Serous Cavity Fluid and Cerebrospinal Fluid Cytopathology

For further volumes:
http://www.springer.com/series/6996

Syed Z. Ali

Department of Pathology, The Johns Hopkins Hospital,
Baltimore, MD, USA

Edmund S. Cibas

Department of Pathology, Brigham and Women's Hospital,
Harvard Medical School, Boston, MA, USA

Serous Cavity Fluid and Cerebrospinal Fluid Cytopathology

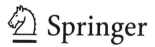

Springer

Syed Z. Ali
Department of Pathology
The Johns Hopkins Hospital
600 N. Wolfe Street
Baltimore, MD 21287, USA
sali@jhmi.edu

Edmund S. Cibas
Department of Pathology
Brigham and Women's Hospital
Harvard Medical School
75 Francis Street
Boston, MA 02115, USA
ecibas@partners.org

ISSN 1574-9053   e-ISSN 1574-9061
ISBN 978-1-4614-1775-0   e-ISBN 978-1-4614-1776-7
DOI 10.1007/978-1-4614-1776-7
Springer New York Dordrecht Heidelberg London

Library of Congress Control Number: 2011943105

Printed on acid-free paper

Springer is part of Springer Science+Business Media (www.springer.com)

Foreword

Serous cavity and cerebrospinal spinal fluids are among the most challenging areas in the practice of cytopathology. Familiarity with the variety of cytomorphological features of specific conditions, along with awareness of the overlapping features of some benign and malignant diseases, is essential to meet these challenges.

In this book, the authors provide a comprehensive yet concise presentation of the cytomorphology and differential diagnoses of various conditions as well as the ancillary techniques which help to establish an accurate diagnosis. A brief description of clinical features and preparation techniques, the basic requirements for an optimal cytopathologic diagnosis, are also included.

The cytopathology of serous cavity fluids is presented in nine chapters. Emphasis is placed on areas of potential diagnostic problems. Ample clinical information is given, as is detailed cytomorphological features for each disease. The current role of immunostains in cytopathologic diagnosis is discussed in detail. Other ancillary techniques, such as flow cytometry, are also presented in appropriate areas.

The other chapter, "Cerebrospinal Fluids," follows the same format. The cytomorphology of metastatic malignant neoplasms and their differential diagnoses are presented in detail. A comprehensive discussion of lymphomas and leukemias includes their cytomorphology, clinical presentation, and differential diagnosis.

Of particular interest, some of the primary central nervous system tumors which are rarely encountered in general practice are presented. Extensive references are provided.

This book should be of great value to practitioners of cytopathology for establishing the diagnosis in challenging cases.

Yener S. Erozan, M.D.
Baltimore, MD, USA
yerozan@jhmi.edu

Series Preface

The subspeciality of cytopathology is 60 years old and has become established as a solid and reliable discipline in medicine. As expected, cytopathology literature has expanded in a remarkably short period of time, from a few textbooks prior to the 1980s to a current and substantial library of texts and journals devoted exclusively to cytomorphology. *Essentials in Cytopathology* does not presume to replace any of the distinguished textbooks in cytopathology. Instead, the series will publish generously illustrated and user-friendly guides for both pathologists and clinicians.

Building on the amazing success of *The Bethesda System for Reporting Cervical Cytology*, now in its second edition, the *Series* will utilize a similar format, including minimal text, tabular criteria, and superb illustrations based on real-life specimens. *Essentials in Cytopathology* will, at times, deviate from the classic organization of pathology texts. The logic of decision trees, elimination of unlikely choices, and narrowing of differential diagnosis via a pragmatic approach based on morphologic criteria will be some of the strategies used to illustrate principles and practice in cytopathology.

Most of the authors for *Essentials in Cytopathology* are faculty members in The Johns Hopkins University School of Medicine, Department of Pathology, Division of Cytopathology. They bring to each volume the legacy of John K. Frost and the collective experience of a preeminent cytopathology service. The archives at Hopkins are meticulously catalogued and form the framework for text and illustrations. Authors from other institutions have been selected on the basis of their national reputations, experience, and enthusiasm for cytopathology. They bring to the series complementary viewpoints and enlarge the scope of materials contained in the photographs.

The editor and authors are indebted to our students, past and future, who challenge and motivate us to become the best that we possibly can be. We share that experience with you through these pages, and hope that you will learn from them as we have from those who have come before us. We would be remiss if we did not pay tribute to our professional colleagues, the cytotechnologists and preparatory technicians who lovingly care for the specimens that our clinical colleagues send to us.

And finally, we cannot emphasize enough throughout these volumes the importance of collaboration with the patient-care team. Every specimen comes to us as a question begging an answer. Without input from the clinicians, complete patient history, results of imaging studies, and other ancillary tests, we cannot perform optimally. It is our responsibility to educate our clinicians about their role in our interpretation, and for us to integrate as much information as we can gather into our final diagnosis, even if the answer at first seems obvious.

We hope you will find this series useful and welcome your feedback as you place these handbooks by your microscopes, and into your book bags.

Dorothy L. Rosenthal
Baltimore MD, USA
drosenthal@jhmi.edu

Contents

1
Introduction, Clinical and Technical Aspects

Background

The three major cavities in the body, that is, pleural, pericardial, and peritoneal, are lined by the serous (or serosal) membrane (and hence the name "serous cavity"). The basic integral component of serosal membrane is a mesothelial cell which loosely rests on submesothelial stromal matrix tissue. These three cavities normally contain a small amount of thin fluid (serous fluid), which helps lubricate the membranes when they rub against each other, such as during breathing, etc. However, in pathologic states, the serous cavities develop spontaneous effusions due to a variety of etiologies. This provides a clinically useful specimen for cytologic evaluation to diagnose the underlying pathologic process, such as infections, inflammation, neoplasia, etc.

In addition to spontaneous effusion, in many patients the serosal membranes (usually abdominal/pelvic) are lavaged with saline and submitted for cytologic analysis to better define the clinical stage in the patient if malignant cells are observed. Cytologic diagnosis by examination of exfoliated cells in serous cavity effusions is one of the most challenging areas in clinical cytopathology. Almost 20% of the effusions examined are directly or indirectly related to the presence of malignant disease, with carcinoma of the lung as the most common underlying culprit. It is easy to understand the

S.Z. Ali and E.S. Cibas, *Serous Cavity Fluid and Cerebrospinal Fluid Cytopathology*, Essentials in Cytopathology 10, DOI 10.1007/ 978-1-4614-1776-7_1, © Springer Science+Business Media, LLC 2012

exfoliation of malignant cells from malignant mesothelioma, the primary cancer of serosal membranes. However, various pathogenetic mechanisms have been suggested when cancer cells involve serous fluids from a distant cancer (see tables below).

Malignant Pleural Effusion – Pathogenesis

- Tumor obstruction of lymphatic flow
- Spread of malignant cells via systemic circulation
- Tumor invasion of pulmonary arterioles

Malignant Neoplasms in Serous Cavity Fluids

- Malignant mesothelioma (epithelioid type)
- Metastatic neoplasms

  - Adenocarcinoma
  - Squamous cell carcinoma
  - Small-cell carcinoma
  - Malignant lymphoma
  - Malignant melanoma
  - Other cancers

Malignant Pleural Effusion – Prognosis

- Median survival following diagnosis – 3–12 months
- Dependent on the stage and type of underlying malignancy
- Shortest survival time – malignant effusions secondary to lung cancer
- Longest survival time – ovarian cancer
- Malignant effusions due to an unknown primary – intermediate survival time

Technical Aspects

Proper collection of serous cavity effusion or washing whether at the patient's bedside or in radiology, and subsequent processing of the specimens and clinical information are prime factors of paramount importance affecting the accuracy of a cytologic diagnosis. Some of the common interpretive problems are created by improper handling of the specimen or lack of the patient's clinical data and radiologic information. Serous cavity fluids (SCF) can be transported to the cytology laboratory in both unfixed and fixed states; we prefer the former. Unfixed (fresh) fluid should be sent to the laboratory as soon as possible. If a delay is expected, the specimen can be kept in the refrigerator. Cell degeneration occurs more rapidly in effusions with extensive acute inflammation and/or blood. Other fluids, however, can be refrigerated for a longer period of time (e.g., overnight, or even over a weekend) without significant loss of cytomorphologic details. Unfixed fluids should be collected in bottles containing 3 units of heparin per milliliter of the estimated fluid to be collected. During collection, the bottle is gently agitated to assure mixture of heparin and fluid. Heparin prevents clotting and therefore trapping of cells in the clot. Fixation of the fluid before transportation may be preferred under certain circumstances (e.g., consistently long delays in transportation). Fifty percent ethanol is usually used for fixation of fluids.

There are various techniques for preparing SCF for cytopathologic examination. Selection of the technique usually depends on the preference of the pathologist, cytotechnologist, work volume, availability of technical personnel, and other factors such as space and cost. As mentioned above, we prefer fresh (unfixed) fluid collected in heparinized containers. From this specimen, cytospin or monolayered preps and paraffin cell blocks are made. Any or all of these preparations depending on the availability can be employed for further special studies, such as immunoperoxidase staining. Therefore, in the presence of an unusual clinical history such as childhood neoplasms, small round blue cell tumors (in any age group), sarcomas, or lymphoproliferative disorders, special precautions should be taken to procure and transport SCF immediately. This is of paramount importance, since a decision can then be made to carry out a variety of ancillary studies, and the portions of the specimen can thus be allocated such as for flow cytometric analysis, molecular testing, etc. Cytospin and cell block preparations can be used for special staining procedures such as mucicarmine and stains for microorganisms and immunocytochemistry. For routine cytology, all prepared slides are fixed in 95% ethanol and stained with Papanicolaou stain. Most prefer not to use air-dried Diff-Quik-stained smears as they are in general considered difficult to interpret and offer no advantage over Papanicolaou-stained smears. Sections of cell block are stained with H & E. If a cell block cannot be prepared from the specimen, two extra cytospin slides are prepared and kept unstained for possible special stains or immunocytochemistry. The importance of proper preparation and staining of cytologic material cannot be overemphasized. Whichever technique is employed, it is essential to strive for high-quality preparations with good cell preservation and staining. There are no clearly defined outlines for specimen adequacy in terms of the quantity of the fluid. However, a minimum of at least 30–50 ml of the fluid should be examined. Some advocate using liquid-based cytology to replace other forms of sample preparation for enhanced quality and diminished false negative rates. Others have concluded that ultrafast Papanicolaou stain improves the resolution of cytoplasmic and nuclear details of nonhematopoietic cells in body fluids for enhanced diagnosis of malignant cells.

Adequate clinical information, including the clinical impression and pertinent radiologic findings, should be stated on the requisition form, which is filled out by the patient's primary physician. Personal contact with the clinician when diagnostic problems arise can certainly be helpful. Some of these problems can be solved after evaluating all available data with the clinician. Specific problems in cytopathologic diagnosis may vary somewhat according to the body site (i.e., pleural, pericardial, and peritoneal cavities), but the problems mentioned at the beginning of this discussion are applicable to all sites.

Ancillary Techniques for the Diagnosis of Serous Cavity Fluids

Serous cavity fluids (SCFs) offer a great sample for almost all routinely performed tests in an anatomic pathology laboratory, ranging from basic enzyme chemistry to more elaborate molecular analyses for a higher accuracy and specific characterization of the pathologic process. Most of these tests will be discussed in appropriate places in the book while discussing more specific disease entities.

- Enzyme cytochemical stains
- Immunoperoxidase stains
- Flow cytometry
- Electron microscopy
- Lipoprotein electrophoresis/serological and chemical analysis, microbiology culture
- Molecular analysis and tumor cytogenetics

Proper collection, preservation, and transportation of the specimen are crucial for ancillary studies performed to supplement a cytomorphologic diagnosis. The ancillary techniques that are often employed in the study of SCF can be categorized into the following general groups:

1. Enzyme cytochemical staining – mucicarmine, PAS with and without diastase digestion, Alcian Blue with and without hyaluronidase treatment, Oil Red O, special stains for microorganisms (Gram, AFB, GMS, PAS, and Gram Weigert stains)
2. Immunoperoxidase labeling – cytokeratins AE1/AE3, CK7, CK20, CK5/6, mCEA, Leu M1, Ber-EP4, calretinin, p53, and other tissue-specific immunomarkers

Cytochemical Stains

- Mucicarmine
- PAS, D-PAS
- Alcian Blue, Alcian Blue with hyaluronidase
- Colloidal iron
- Oil Red O

Immunoperoxidase (IPOX) Stains

- Mesothelioma vs. adenocarcinoma markers
- Organ-specific markers
- Tissue-specific markers
- Others

Diagnostic Profile

Most patients with suspected cancers or known malignancies routinely undergo cytologic evaluation of SCFs. Cytologic examination of SCFs is an extremely useful diagnostic procedure, which helps define the clinical stage of patients with oncologic disease. Overall considered to be a highly accurate diagnostic procedure, cytologic evaluation of SCFs has been reported to have a high specificity but low to moderate sensitivity for detecting malignant cells. The following table summarizes the overall figures as published in major series on this subject:

- Sensitivity   50–62.4%
- Specificity   97%
- PPV   95.7–100%
- NPV   86.4–88.3%

As can be seen above, the reported lower sensitivity is a controversial issue as in most cases of SCFs, which are reported cytologically benign, there are no "gold standard" follow-up tissue studies of the serosa available to calculate the true or false negativity of a cytologic assessment. Additionally, a mere positive follow-up biopsy or repeat fluid analysis with malignant cells at a later stage does not constitute a previous effusion being false negative. One study (Hsu) has the sensitivity of cytologic detection to be 6.7% higher than that of pleural biopsy, the cytopathologic correlation to be 96.5% accurate, with 0.1% false-positive results and 0.18% false-negative results by cytology.

Major Diagnostic Issues in Cytologic Interpretation of Serous Cavity Fluids

Cytologic interpretation of SCFs is often diagnostically challenging. There are at least six main reasons for the above fact:

- SCFs commonly contain abundant reactive mesothelial cells, histiocytes, and lymphocytes. If the effusion contains rare malignant cells, those are often obscured by the relative overabundance of these other cellular elements and hence may not be readily detectable on microscopic examination.
- Malignant cells are often exfoliated as single cells or minute tissue fragments if the sample being examined is a spontaneous effusion (such as ascitic fluid). Thus, a relative lack of cellular architecture may hamper an accurate cytologic assessment.
- Neoplastic cells may significantly "morph" and change their appearance by being suspended in serous fluids for a prolonged period of time after being exfoliated. Cells may appear more rounded and cytoplasm may develop pseudo vacuoles, and, therefore, most of their morphologic "kinship" to the primary tumor could be lost.
- Quite often, at the time of cytologic evaluation, there is no known history of a prior malignancy available ("occult metastasis") or the patient may have more than one known cancer, and determining the primary cancer based on SCF analysis becomes a challenging task.
- A cytomorphologic distinction between reactive mesothelial cells, malignant mesothelioma, and metastatic adenocarcinoma can often be extremely difficult due to significant morphologic overlap.
- Malignant mesothelioma is potentially a litigation diagnosis due to its strong association with industrial exposure to asbestos. Therefore, such diagnosis in SCF has to be made with careful evaluation, supported by an adequate number of immunostains. The latter can become a difficult issue in a limited cytologic specimen.

"Effusion = Confusion"

The following table summarizes the outline followed in this monograph for a practical approach to selected diagnostically difficult areas of SCF interpretation:

- Reactive mesothelial hyperplasia vs. malignant mesothelioma
- Malignant mesothelioma vs. metastatic adenocarcinoma
- Nonepithelial, nonmesothelial malignancies mimicking adenocarcinoma
- Sarcomatous effusions
- Effusions in children
- Determining primary site of a metastatic carcinoma
- Lymphoid-rich effusions

Selected Reading

Ceelen GH. The cytologic diagnosis of ascitic fluid. Symp Diagn Accuracy Cytol Techn. 1964;8:175–85.

Davidson B. Malignant effusions: from diagnosis to biology. Diagn Cytopathol. 2004;31(4):246–54.

Gabriel C, Achten R, Drijkoningen M. Use of liquid-based cytology in serous fluids: a comparison with conventional cytopreparatory techniques. Acta Cytol. 2004;48(6):825–35.

Grunze H. The comparative diagnostic accuracy, efficiency and specificity of cytologic techniques used in the diagnosis of malignant neoplasm in serous effusions of the pleural and pericardial cavities. Acta Cytol. 1964;8:150–63.

Hsu C. Cytologic detection of malignancy in pleural effusion: a review of 5,255 samples from 3,811 patients. Diagn Cytopathol. 1987;3(1):8–12.

Johnson WD. The cytological diagnosis of cancer in serous effusions. Acta Cytol. 1966;10:161–72.

Lopez Cardozo P. A critical evaluation of 3,000 cytologic analyses of pleural fluid, ascitic fluid and pericardial fluid. Acta Cytol. 1966;10:455–60.

Motherby H, Nadjari B, Friegel P, Kohaus J, Ramp U, Böcking A. Diagnostic accuracy of effusion cytology. Diagn Cytopathol. 1999;20:350–7.

Nance KV, Shermer RW, Askin FB. Diagnostic efficacy of pleural biopsy as compared with that of pleural fluid examination. Mod Pathol. 1991;4: 320–4.

Naylor B, Schmidt RW. The case for exfoliative cytology of serous effusions. Lancet. 1964;1:711–2.

Ueda J, Iwata T, Ono M, Takahashi M. Comparison of three cytologic preparation methods and immunocytochemistries to distinguish adenocarcinoma cells from reactive mesothelial cells in serous effusion. Diagn Cytopathol. 2006;34(1):6–10.

Yang GC, Papellas J, Wu HC, Waisman J. Application of Ultrafast Papanicolaou stain to body fluid cytology. Acta Cytol. 2001;45(2):180–5.

2
Normal Cytology

Major Cell Types Commonly Seen in SCFs (Figs. 2.1 and 2.2)

- Histiocytes
- Lymphomononuclear cells
- Mesothelial cells
- Other cells (red blood cells, PMNs)

Histiocytes (Figs. 2.3 and 2.4)

These cells predominate in any type of SCF (with the exception of abdominopelvic surgical washings). The histiocytes are large cells with a round central nucleus and an ample amount of often finely vacuolated cytoplasm. The nucleus may contain a prominent nucleolus. A key feature is the presence of well-defined cytoplasm. Macrophages are typically seen singly. However, when a large volume effusion is concentrated in the laboratory, the macrophages may significantly overlap and may give a false impression of true tissue fragments.

S.Z. Ali and E.S. Cibas, *Serous Cavity Fluid and Cerebrospinal Fluid Cytopathology*, Essentials in Cytopathology 10, DOI 10.1007/ 978-1-4614-1776-7_2, © Springer Science+Business Media, LLC 2012

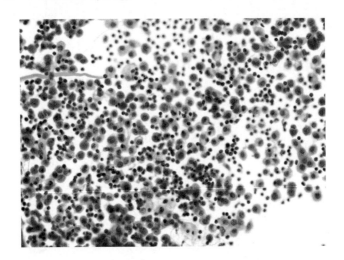

FIG. 2.1. *Benign SCF.* Note the polymorphous mixture of a variety of cell types at low magnification. These are predominantly reactive mesothelial cells, histiocytes, and lymphocytes (Papanicolaou, low power).

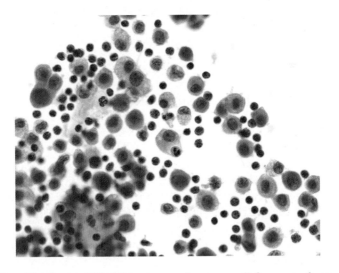

FIG. 2.2. *Benign SCF.* Higher power shows a small fragment of mesothelial cells at 10 o'clock in a background of abundant histiocytes, lymphocytes, and PMNs. Mesothelial cells and histiocytes are almost the same size, and occasionally an adequate distinction cannot be made between the two cell types (Papanicolaou, high power).

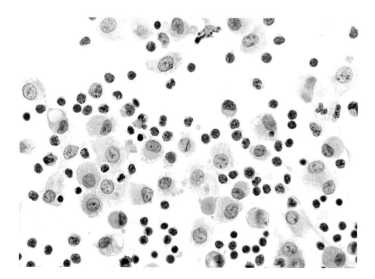

FIG. 2.3. *Histiocytes in benign SCF.* These are larger cells with abundant finely vacuolated cytoplasm and large central or eccentric nucleus with or without a small nucleolus. Mesothelial cells may also occasionally develop cytoplasmic vacuolization as a degenerative change. Note the background lymphomononuclear cells (Papanicolaou, high power).

Lymphomononuclear Cells

These are easy to recognize in any effusion specimen. They are small with a round nucleus, inconspicuous nucleolus, and scant cytoplasm. Most cells appear as naked nuclei and are intimately admixed with histiocytes and mesothelial cells. In general, lymphocytes, when present in abundance, should show a variation in size (polymorphism) and be of predominantly T-cell lineage. More details are included in a separate chapter later in the book.

Mesothelial Cells (Figs. 2.5, 2.6 and 2.7)

Mesothelial cells are typically singly dispersed among histiocytes and lymphocytes. They are large cells (15–20 mm) with a centrally placed large nucleus often displaying an inconspicuous single nucleolus. Their cytoplasm often appears denser in comparison to

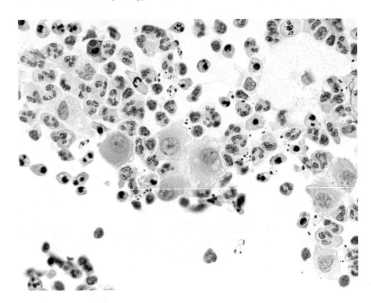

Fig. 2.4. *Histiocytes and PMNs.* Note the finely vacuolated cytoplasm of the histiocytes. The two cells at 3 o'clock have cytoplasmic vacuolization, but their two-cell relationship suggests a mesothelial origin. In such case, an accurate distinction can be difficult. In general, mesothelial cells have a denser (more opaque) cytoplasm. However, degenerated single mesothelial cells can be extremely difficult to distinguish from histiocytes (Papanicolaou, high power).

the histiocytes, but, commonly due to degenerative changes, the cells may show prominent vacuolization. In the latter case, a morphological distinction with the background histiocytes may not be always possible. Occasionally, mesothelial cells can be observed in small fragments of 2 to 6 cells. Larger benign-appearing fragments are usually a sign of reactive hyperplasia and rarely a well-differentiated mesothelioma. The outer border of mesothelial cells may appear "fuzzy" due to the presence of bundles of long and floppy microvilli. This cytologic feature is accentuated more in reactive mesothelial hyperplasia and malignant mesothelioma creating the so-called "lacy border" or "cytoplasmic whiskers" better seen on Diff-Quik or ultrafast Papanicolaou stains. When seen closer to each other, adjacent cells may be separated by a small ill-defined clear zone referred to as a "cell window."

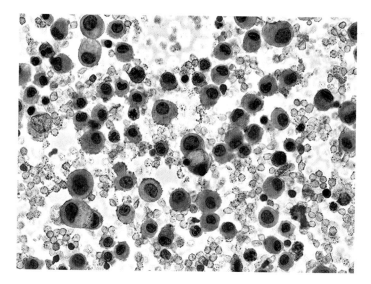

Fɪɢ. 2.5. *Mesothelial cells.* This field predominantly shows mesothelial cells with the characteristic denser or opaque cytoplasm, large nucleus, small nucleolus, and lack of cytoplasmic vacuolization. Doublets (or groups of two cells) with the diagnostic intercellular "window" make identification quite straightforward in such cases (Papanicolaou, high power).

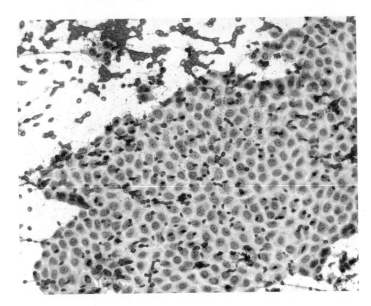

Fig. 2.6. *Mesothelial cells.* A large monolayered sheet of benign mesothelial cells is seen here. Note the cellular monotony and a "tissue culture"–type appearance caused by fragile wispy cytoplasmic junctions between adjacent cells. Large tissue fragments are highly unusual in a spontaneous effusion and are almost always obtained during an intraoperative peritoneal washing (Papanicolaou, low power).

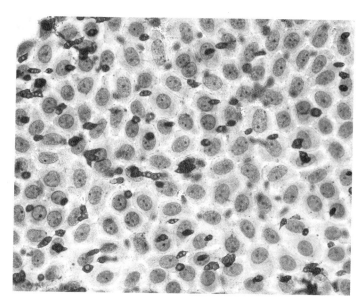

FIG. 2.7. *Mesothelial cells.* Higher magnification shows large round to oval uniform nuclei, pale nuclear chromatin, small nucleoli, and fairly distinct intercellular spaces or "windows" (Papanicolaou, high power).

3
Reactive Mesothelial Hyperplasia

This condition often accompanies certain specific underlying medical conditions. However, in a large number of cases, no apparent cause can be assigned to the presence of reactive mesothelial hyperplasia (RMH) in an effusion specimen. Common causes of florid mesothelial hyperplasia include ischemic conditions of heart and lung (pulmonary infarction being the most notorious cause), systemic diseases (collagen-vascular diseases, SLE, etc.), hepatic cirrhosis, infections, radiation therapy, and underlying malignancy.

Clinico-Cytopathologic Characteristics (Figs. 3.1, 3.2, 3.3, 3.4, 3.5, 3.6, 3.7, 3.8, 3.9, 3.10, 3.11 and 3.12)

- Most common cause – ischemic conditions (CHF, pulmonary infarct)
- Hypercellular specimen
- Predominantly single cells
- Cell aggregates and small tissue fragments, mostly doublets and rarely in fragments with 2–6 cells

(continued)

S.Z. Ali and E.S. Cibas, *Serous Cavity Fluid and Cerebrospinal Fluid Cytopathology*, Essentials in Cytopathology 10, DOI 10.1007/ 978-1-4614-1776-7_3, © Springer Science+Business Media, LLC 2012

- Few papillary tissue fragments
- Single cells or cells in aggregates may vary in size and N/C ratio
- Nuclei usually round and centrally located
- Chromatin texture varies but usually evenly dispersed
- Nucleoli, single or multiple, can become prominent
- Background: histiocytes and inflammatory cells (often mixed type) in varying numbers

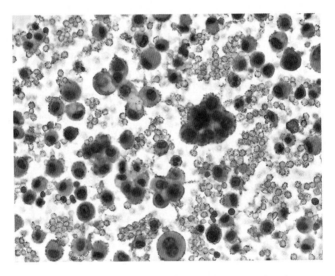

FIG. 3.1. *Reactive mesothelial hyperplasia.* Abundance of benign-appearing mesothelial cells, seen singly and in small tissue fragments. Lack of cytologic atypia (high N/C ratios, hyperchromasia, macronucleoli, and binucleation) distinguishes these cells from malignant mesothelioma (Papanicolaou, high power).

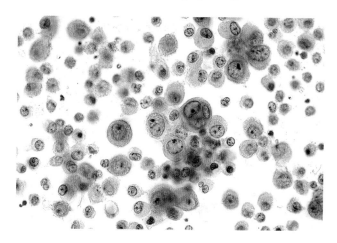

FIG. 3.2. *Reactive mesothelial hyperplasia with atypia.* Initial impression in this pleural effusion was a malignant mesothelioma because of hypercellularity caused by these atypical-appearing mesothelial cells with occasional prominent nucleoli, binucleation/multinucleation, and intact (although small) tissue fragments. However, the patient was a 21-year-old pregnant woman who had symptoms of pelvic thrombophlebitis and breathing difficulties and was found to have a pulmonary infarct (Papanicolaou, high power).

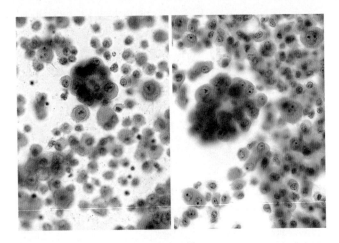

FIG. 3.3. *Reactive mesothelial hyperplasia with marked cytologic atypia.* Note the intact tissue fragments with cells forming "acini"-like structures. Cells have large nuclei, high N/C ratios, and prominent nucleoli. A careful correlation with patient's clinical history, presenting complaints, and radiologic findings is crucial to avoid an overcall (Papanicolaou, high power).

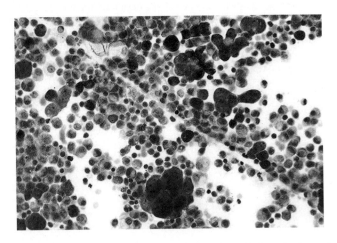

FIG. 3.4. *Reactive mesothelial hyperplasia with marked cytologic atypia.* Diff-Quik-stained SCF smears are the most difficult to interpret. Presence of numerous tissue fragments and cells with macronucleoli makes the interpretation of this case particularly challenging (Diff-Quik, high power).

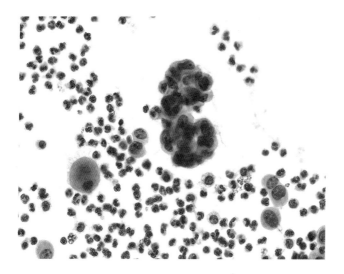

FIG. 3.5. *Reactive mesothelial hyperplasia with marked cytologic atypia.* Acute serositis resulted in exfoliation of numerous tissue fragments of mesothelial cells with high N/C ratios and discrete macronucleoli. In such cases a repeat tap and cytology after treatment may result in disappearance of the cytologic atypia. History of an underlying pathologic process (such as SLE) would be extremely helpful for an accurate cytologic interpretation (Papanicolaou, high power).

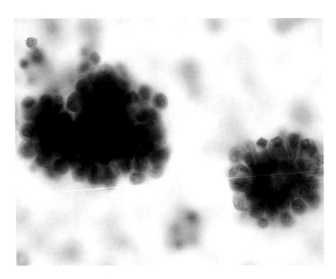

FIG. 3.6. *Reactive mesothelial hyperplasia.* Large tissue fragments of mesothelial cells presenting a "papillary-like" configuration. A well-differentiated mesothelioma would be hard to exclude in such cases. These intact fragments are much more often associated with reactive hyperplasia in patients with benign gynecologic tract diseases (such as endometriosis) and are almost always seen in abdominopelvic washings, as in this particular case (Papanicolaou, high power).

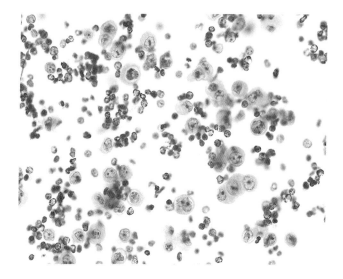

FIG. 3.7. *Reactive mesothelial hyperplasia.* Numerous mesothelial cells are seen in a background of lymphomononuclear cells. The mesothelial cells show atypia with high N/C ratios, irregular nuclear membranes, hyperchromasia, and prominent nucleoli. Few intact tissue fragments are also visible (Papanicolaou, high power).

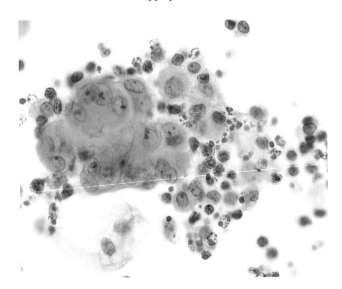

FIG. 3.8. *Reactive mesothelial hyperplasia.* A large tissue fragment of hyperplastic mesothelium is seen here. Note the nuclear irregularity and occasional prominent nucleoli. A metastatic adenocarcinoma will also be high on the list of differential diagnoses. Such cases often need confirmatory immunostaining (Papanicolaou, high power).

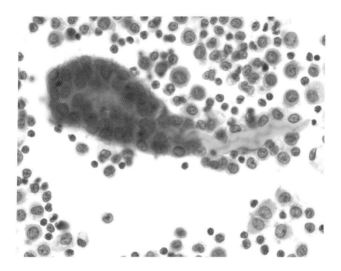

FIG. 3.9. *Reactive mesothelial hyperplasia.* This patient with advanced hepatic cirrhosis repeatedly developed large-volume abdominal effusions containing fragments of atypical mesothelium. Along with pulmonary infarction, hepatic cirrhosis is a leading cause of "mesothelial atypia" in an effusion specimen. One should have a much higher threshold for malignancy if the patient has known history of these medical conditions. The fragment in this particular case shows the most unusual feature, that is, the presence of a well-formed Herxheimer spiral, a microscopic feature which has been described in benign and malignant squamous cells (Papanicolaou, high power).

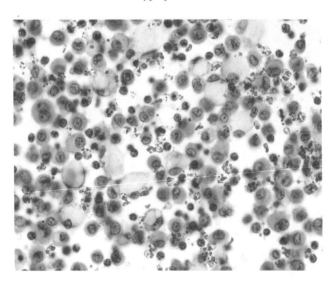

FIG. 3.10. *Reactive mesothelial hyperplasia.* Abdominal fluid with abundant "signet-ring"-type cells containing single large cytoplasmic vacuoles pushing the nucleus to the periphery. The leading cause of "signet-ring" cells in SCF is NOT a metastatic signet-ring cell adenocarcinoma, rather atypical mesothelial hyperplasia in patients with advanced hepatic cirrhosis. These "pseudo signet-ring" cells likely represent degenerative changes as the author has observed this phenomenon numerous times in pleural effusions as well (Papanicolaou, low power).

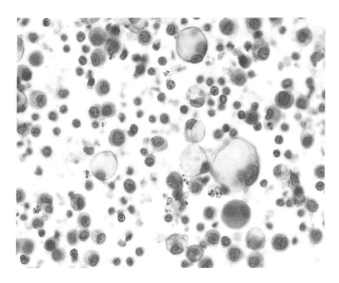

Fɪɢ. 3.11. *Reactive mesothelial hyperplasia.* Higher magnification of another case from a patient with hepatic cirrhosis illustrates the pseudo signet-ring cells (Papanicolaou, high power).

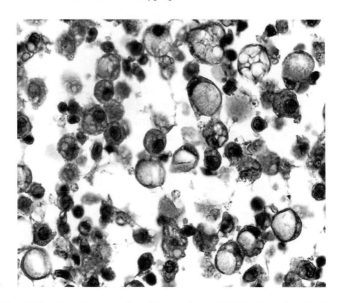

Fig. 3.12. *Reactive mesothelial hyperplasia.* Cell block section displays the well-formed signet-ring cells. A mucicarmine stain would be negative in these cases and will be the simplest way to distinguish these from a true signet-ring cell adenocarcinoma which most often originates in the stomach (H & E, high power).

The morphologic separation of benign reactive and hyperplastic mesothelium from malignant mesothelioma can be a daunting task (Figs. 3.1, 3.2, 3.3, 3.4, 3.5, 3.6, 3.7 and 3.8). In a study of 217 cases that were independently reviewed by members of the US-Canadian Mesothelioma Reference Panel, in approximately 22% of cases there was disagreement on whether the interpretation was benign or malignant. Experts (Churg et al.) have concluded that "labeling an equivocal proliferation atypical mesothelial hyperplasia or a similar term is far better than overdiagnosing a malignancy, because further diagnostic specimens can usually be obtained, and true malignant mesotheliomas make themselves evident, in most cases, in short order." True stromal invasion is considered the most accurate indicator of mesothelial malignancy, a feature often difficult to assess in small biopsies and impossible to ascertain in

SCFs. Presence of cytologic atypia is not helpful in distinguishing benign from malignant reactions, since benign proliferations are commonly atypical and malignant mesotheliomas can often be deceptively monotonous. Therefore, the classic features of malignancy (pleomorphism, high N/C ratios, hyperchromasia, prominent nucleoli, and mitoses) may not be accurate in distinguishing the two groups of lesions. Adequate information of the clinico-radiologic findings (history of asbestos exposure, chronic lung disease, chest pain, pleural-based mass, etc.) is important.

Reactive Mesothelial Hyperplasia vs. Malignant Mesothelioma

- Clinico-radiologic findings
- Cytomorphology
- EMA, desmin, GLUT-1, p53, and other immunomarkers

Florid peritoneal mesothelial hyperplasia is often an accompaniment of various gynecological diseases and may be associated with a variety of benign and malignant entities, the most common of which are endometriosis and endosalpingiosis. These and other entities are presented in a separate chapter later in this book. A prominent papillary-like architecture and numerous psammoma bodies are usually the hallmark of such proliferative processes.

Major Underlying Causes of Mesothelial Proliferation

- Pulmonary infarct[a]
- Heart failure
- Hepatic cirrhosis[a]
- Chronic renal failure (with or without peritoneal dialysis)
- Pancreatitis

(continued)

- Radiation therapy[a]
- Autoimmune disorders (SLE)[a]
- Gynecologic tract diseases (endometriosis, endosalpingiosis, ovarian adenofibroma)
- Post-surgical

Over the years, many immunomarkers have been proposed that have a potential role in making this distinction. Historically, several laboratories have used EMA and desmin. An accurate interpretation of the qualitatively different patterns of staining with EMA in benign versus malignant mesothelium is often quite difficult. Studies have shown that EMA in general is expressed more often in mesothelioma (100%) than in reactive mesothelium. Likewise, desmin is known to be immunoexpressed more often in benign mesothelium (84%) than malignant (6%). GLUT-1, a member of the glucose transporter (GLUT) family of passive carriers, has displayed promising results. It has been shown to be immunoexpressed in 47–100% of mesotheliomas (linear cell membrane staining) and in 0–12% of benign mesothelium.

p53 mutations are common in malignant neoplasms. p53 immunoexpression is highly specific (100%) but suffers from a relatively low sensitivity. The criterion for a truly positive p53 immunostain is hard to define. However, most agree that a few sporadic positive nuclei should be interpreted with caution as positive. Most agree that a strong staining of >10% nuclei constitutes a true positive case.

p53 Immunostaining in Mesothelial Hyperplasia vs. Cancer

- Monoclonal antibody Do-7
- Positivity in malignancy – 32–55%
- None of the benign effusions stain
- Highly specific (100%)
- Moderately sensitive

---

[a]May additionally cause significant cytologic atypia warranting a higher threshold for malignancy when such effusions are examined cytologically

GLUT-1 Immunostaining in Mesothelial Hyperplasia vs. Cancer

- One of the glucose transport proteins found in various human cells
- Normally expressed in human blood-brain barrier, placenta, skin and its adnexae, and erythrocytes
- Displays membranous staining pattern with or without cytoplasmic staining
- Red blood cells stain positively creating interpretation issues in bloody effusions
- Highly specific (88–97%)
- Moderately sensitive (47–60%)

Recently, an insulin-like growth factor II messenger ribonucleic acid-binding protein 3 (IMP3), an oncofetal protein, has been shown to be of value as a biomarker to distinguish between malignant and reactive mesothelial cells when used as an immunohistochemical stain for IMP3 expression. IMP3 showed strong cytoplasmic staining in 73% of mesothelioma cases (in contrast to an undetectable expression in benign reactive mesothelial proliferations).

Pan-cell proliferation markers like Ki-67 have been used either alone or in combination with other antibodies (such as p53). Studies have shown that the mean labeling index for Ki-67 in malignant mesothelioma is around 25% (range, 1–66%) and 6% for benign mesothelial proliferation (range, 0–25%). In our experience, Ki-67 has very limited, if any, value in routine evaluation of SCFs.

HBME-1 is another potential marker that has been used in cytologic smears. Many immunohistochemical studies have concluded that HBME-1 has a high sensitivity (~93%) but a moderate (83%) specificity for benign mesothelial proliferation vs. malignant mesothelioma.

Selected Reading

Churg A, Colby TV, Cagle P, Corson J, Gibbs AR, Gilks B, Grimes M, Hammar S, Roggli V, Travis WD. The separation of benign and malignant mesothelial proliferations. Am J Surg Pathol. 2000;24(9): 1183–200.

Hasteh F, Lin GY, Weidner N, Michael CW. The use of immunohistochemistry to distinguish reactive mesothelial cells from malignant mesothelioma in cytologic effusions. Cancer Cytopathol. 2010;118(2):90–6.

Kato Y, Tsuta K, Seki K, Maeshima AM, Watanabe S, Suzuki K, Asamura H, Tsuchiya R, Matsuno Y. Immunohistochemical detection of GLUT-1 can discriminate between reactive mesothelium and malignant mesothelioma. Mod Pathol. 2007;20(2):215–20.

Malle D, Valeri RM, Photiou C, Kaplanis K, Andreadis C, Tsavdaridis D, Destouni C. Significance of immunocytochemical expression of E-cadherin, N-cadherin and CD44 in serous effusions using liquid-based cytology. Acta Cytol. 2005;49(1):11–6.

Monaco SE, Shuai Y, Bansal M, Krasinskas AM, Dacic S. The diagnostic utility of p16 FISH and GLUT-1 immunohistochemical analysis in mesothelial proliferations. Am J Clin Pathol. 2011;135(4):619–27.

Mullick SS, Green LK, Ramzy I, Brown RW, Smith D, Gondo MM, Cagle PT. p53 gene product in pleural effusions. Practical use in distinguishing benign from malignant cells. Acta Cytol. 1996;40(5):855–60.

Politi E, Kandaraki C, Apostolopoulou C, Kyritsi T, Koutselini H. Immunocytochemical panel for distinguishing between carcinoma and reactive mesothelial cells in body cavity fluids. Diagn Cytopathol. 2005;32(3):151–5.

Sakuma N, Kamei T, Ishihara T. Ultrastructure of pleural mesothelioma and pulmonary adenocarcinoma in malignant effusions as compared with reactive mesothelial cells. Acta Cytol. 1999;43(5):777–85.

Saleh HA, El-Fakharany M, Makki H, Kadhim A, Masood S. Differentiating reactive mesothelial cells from metastatic adenocarcinoma in serous effusions: the utility of immunocytochemical panel in the differential diagnosis. Diagn Cytopathol. 2009;37(5):324–32.

Shen J, Pinkus GS, Deshpande V, Cibas ES. Usefulness of EMA, GLUT-1, and XIAP for the cytologic diagnosis of malignant mesothelioma in body cavity fluids. Am J Clin Pathol. 2009;131(4):516–23.

Su XY, Li GD, Liu WP, Xie B, Jiang YH. Cytological differential diagnosis among adenocarcinoma, epithelial mesothelioma, and reactive mesothelial cells in serous effusions by immunocytochemistry. Diagn Cytopathol. 2011;39(12):900–8.

Zoppi JA, Pellicer EM, Sundblad AS. Diagnostic value of p53 protein in the study of serous effusions. Acta Cytol. 1995;39(4):721–4.

4
Malignant Mesothelioma
"A Potential Litigation Diagnosis"

Malignant mesothelioma (MM) is a rare, high-grade cancer that is directly linked to asbestos exposure. This link between asbestos and MM was first noted in asbestos miners in the 1940s in South Africa. Other documented causes include high-dose radiation exposure, recurrent pleuritis/peritonitis, and infection with simian virus 40 (SV40). Malignant pleural mesothelioma is most common, whereas malignant peritoneal mesothelioma accounts only for 6–10% of all cases. Significantly less common than lung cancer, there are 2,000–3,000 new cases of thoracic MM each year. The gradual increase in the number of newly diagnosed MM is attributed to the widespread use of asbestos as an insulation material in the latter half of the last century (in shipbuilding, pipefitting, and other construction and automobile brakes). The needle-like asbestos fibers escape from the lung into the pleural space, causing chronic irritation and, rarely, malignant transformation in some patients. Asbestos-exposed individuals with radiographic evidence of pleural plaques are at increased risk for lung cancer and pleural mesothelioma, compared to the general population. Often there is a long latency period between exposure and onset of malignant mesothelioma ranging from 15 to 60 years. Thoracic MM is much more common in men (M:F, 13:1) with an average age of 55 years. Chest pain is often the most common symptom. Rarer are other sites of origin: pericardium and tunica vaginalis (1–2%).

S.Z. Ali and E.S. Cibas, *Serous Cavity Fluid and Cerebrospinal Fluid Cytopathology*, Essentials in Cytopathology 10, DOI 10.1007/ 978-1-4614-1776-7_4,

Thoracic MM is radiographically characterized by diffuse asymmetric pleural thickening. MM displays either diffuse growth pattern or occurs as a localized nodular mass. The diffuse-type pleural effusion is present in more than 95% of the cases. MM is more aggressive with poor prognosis and is deemed incurable in most cases. MM shows two major histologic subtypes: epithelioid (more common) and sarcomatoid. Tumors displaying histologic features of both subtypes are often classified into mixed or biphasic variant (accounting for 30% of all cases). Although histological subtyping is an important prognostic marker, it is often not possible to differentiate the subtypes in a limited SCF specimen. In cytologic material from SCFs, the predominant subtype diagnosed is the epithelioid variant. Sarcomatoid MM is uncommon and rarely diagnosed on SCF cytology as its fibrous nature prevents the malignant cells from exfoliating spontaneously. Well-differentiated papillary mesothelioma is generally considered a noninvasive subtype of mesothelioma with low malignant potential that arises mostly in females in the peritoneal cavity. Molecular analyses have identified several oncogenetic pathways that appear activated in MM. Numerous tumor suppressor genes, including p16, p14, and p53, appear involved, and aberrant expression of growth factors/receptors such as TGF-a, PDGF, IGF, and HGF has been implicated. Standard management includes chemotherapy, radiation therapy, and surgical resection (decortication, pleurectomy, or pneumonectomy) with adjuvant therapy. Most patients have an average survival posttreatment of 10.5 months with an average 5-year survival rate of less than 9%. Patients with sarcomatoid histology had worse prognosis than patients with epithelioid and biphasic histological subtypes.

The days of the older medical literature claiming that the diagnosis of malignant mesothelioma can only be rendered at autopsy are long gone. However, malignant mesothelioma is a serious diagnosis and should be carefully rendered after considering patient's clinical history (asbestos exposure), radiologic findings, cytomorphologic features, and immunostaining profile. Patients with MM commonly develop spontaneous effusions that tend to recur after initial tapping. Most often SCFs in patients with MM will contain a large amount of malignant cells with well-developed cytomorphologic characteristics. However, diagnostic issues arise when the amount of lesional cells is low or when cytomorphology overlaps significantly with metastatic adenocarcinoma (a common scenario).

- Clinico-radiologic findings
- Cytomorphologic characteristics
- Enzyme cytochemical staining
- Immunoperoxidase studies

Etiologic Factors

- Occupational or paraoccupational exposure to asbestos (strongest association present in 90% of patients) or erionite. All types of asbestos fibers can cause mesothelioma, although crocidolite is considered a higher risk with a dose-related effect
- Irradiation
- Simian virus 40 (SV40) infection
- Genetic predisposition
- Chronic inflammation due to exposure to other chemicals

Clinico-Radiologic Features

- Incidence increases with age (10 times higher in men aged 60–64 years than in those aged 30–34)
- Insiduous onset
- Usually a long latency period
- In pleural disease – chest pain, dyspnea and/or cough, pleural/pericardial effusions, dysphagia, weight loss, night sweats
- In peritoneal disease – nausea and vomiting, abdominal pain and distension, recurrent ascites, bowel obstruction, abdominal and pelvic masses, obstructive uropathy
- Chest radiographs – unilateral pleural abnormalities with effusions
- CT scans – encapsulation of the lung by thickened pleura

Therapeutic Approach and Prognostic Outcomes

- Chemotherapy, surgery, and radiotherapy – variable effect
- Chemotherapy – useful in palliation and can improve both survival and quality of life
- Role of radical surgery yet unclear
- Multimodality treatments appear to be the most successful
- Novel therapies – intrapleural chemotherapy, photodynamic therapy, and hyperthermic perfusion
- Immunomodulation and targeted treatments are being developed
  - Inhibitors of epidermal growth factor receptor (EGFR), vascular endothelial growth factor (VEGF), and histone deacetylases
  - Antibodies against VEGFR and mesothelin
- Aggressive and rapidly fatal
- Median survival of 8 months for untreated cases
- Two years or longer survival when surgery is combined with adjuvant therapy (selected cases)

Malignant Mesothelioma (Epithelioid type) (Figs. 4.1, 4.2, 4.3, 4.4, 4.5, 4.6, 4.7, 4.8, 4.9, 4.10, 4.11, 4.12, 4.13, 4.14, 4.15, 4.16, 4.17, 4.18, 4.19, 4.20, 4.21, 4.22 and 4.23)

- *Cytomorphologic features* Hypercellular smears with a mostly "one-cell" population
  - Single cells and tissue fragments (three-dimensional balls, papillary-like branching fragments)
  - Usually large cells with prominent nucleoli
  - Malignant features such as sharp irregularities of nuclear contour, irregular chromatin distribution (present in poorly differentiated tumors, may be subtle or absent in well-differentiated mesothelioma)

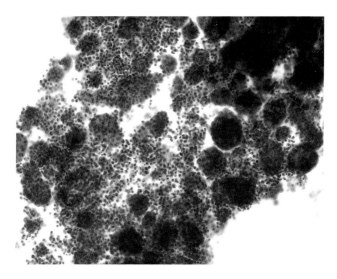

FIG. 4.1. *Malignant mesothelioma.* This hypercellular picture consists of cells in fragments as well as abundant singly dispersed cells. The three-dimensional tissue fragments have an acinus-like architecture. Hypercellularity is a common feature, and the amount of neoplastic cells is mostly higher compared with metastatic cancers in SCF (Papanicolaou, low power).

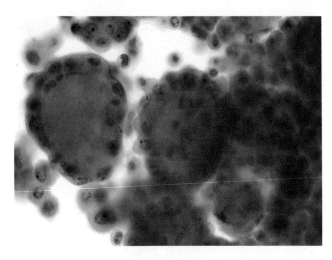

Fig. 4.2. *Malignant mesothelioma.* Higher magnification reveals the acinus-like architecture, with a pale green core surrounded by a layer of malignant cells. Note the undulating outer border of the cell fragments which would be in sharp contrast to a much smoother outline of adeno-carcinoma fragments (examples shown in Chap. 5) (Papanicolaou, high power).

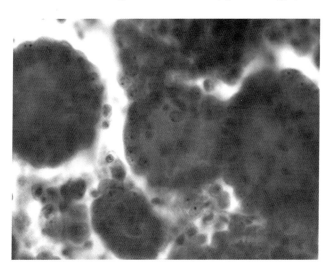

FIG. 4.3. *Malignant mesothelioma.* Another view illustrates the three dimensionality of the cellular fragments. Nuclei are round with prominent nucleoli. The center of these cellular fragments consists of loose submesothelial matrix tissue which appears pale green on Papanicolaou stain (Papanicolaou, high power).

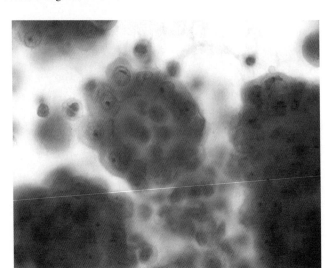

FIG. 4.4. *Malignant mesothelioma.* Pictured is a gland-like fragment of malignant cells with the characteristic "hob-nailed" appearance of the outer border due to prominence of the large nuclei. Also seen here are single discrete macronucleoli. Most metastatic adenocarcinomas tend to have a smooth outer contour in the exfoliated tissue fragments (Papanicolaou, high power).

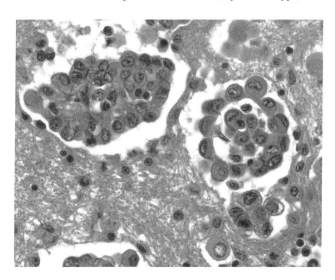

Fɪɢ. 4.5. *Malignant mesothelioma.* Cell block section displays gland-like fragments comprised of cells with enlarged nuclei containing macronucleoli. The central portion of the cellular fragments likely contains matrix tissue with embedded cells (as opposed to mucin which is seen in metastatic adenocarcinomas) (H & E, high power).

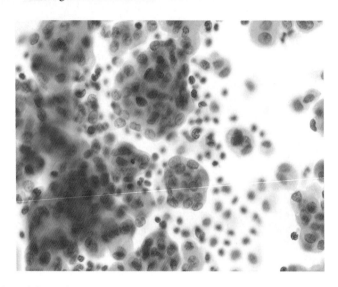

FIG. 4.6. *Malignant mesothelioma.* Numerous malignant cells in three-dimensional balls and irregular crowded tissue fragments are seen. A distinction from adenocarcinoma may require immunostaining for a definitive diagnosis (Papanicolaou, high power).

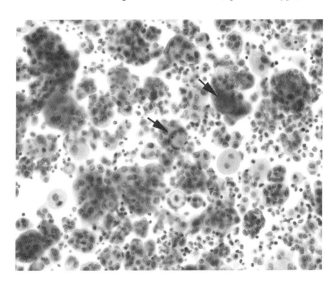

FIG. 4.7. *Malignant mesothelioma.* This was an extremely cellular smear comprised of nearly all malignant cells. Malignant mesothelioma may occasionally demonstrate well-formed intracytoplasmic vacuoles containing acidic mucin. This can create diagnostic confusion with metastatic mucin-producing adenocarcinoma. A mucicarmine stain or PAS with and without diastase digestion can confirm the specific nature of the mucin (as being acidic or mesenchymal-type in mesothelioma compared to the neutral mucin of an adenocarcinoma) (Papanicolaou, low power).

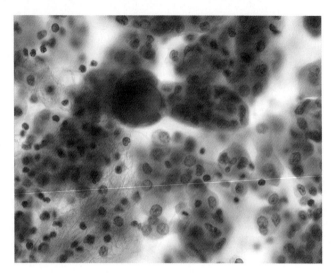

Fɪɢ. 4.8. *Malignant mesothelioma.* A higher magnification nicely illustrates a large intracytoplasmic mucin vacuole. Smear background also appears to contain pale pink mucinous matrix material. The possibility of a mucin-producing adenocarcinoma should be carefully excluded in such instances. In these cases of mesothelioma, the gross appearance of the effusion fluid may assume a thick "honey-like" consistency due to large amount of acidic mucin/matrix and hyaluronic acid (Papanicolaou, high power).

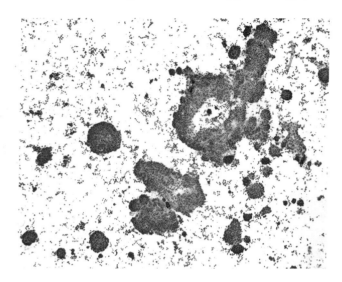

FIG. 4.9. *Malignant mesothelioma.* Diff-Quik stain is uncommonly done in SCFs. In this smear, the malignant cells are seen primarily as three-dimensional ball-like fragments and irregular sheets. The differential diagnostic considerations in this case would include severe mesothelial hyperplasia and a metastatic adenocarcinoma (Diff-Quik, low power).

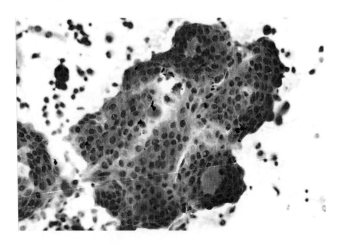

FIG. 4.10. *Malignant mesothelioma.* Higher magnification of a cellular fragment from the previous case illustrates three dimensionality, cytoplasmic opacity, and pale magenta–colored stroma in the middle of a cell ball (Diff-Quik, high power).

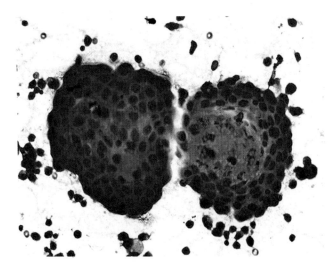

FIG. 4.11. *Malignant mesothelioma.* This is a better illustration of the three-dimensional architecture of the malignant cellular fragments. Notice the irregular undulating outer border with the center of the fragment containing pale magenta–colored submesothelial matrix tissue (Diff-Quik, high power).

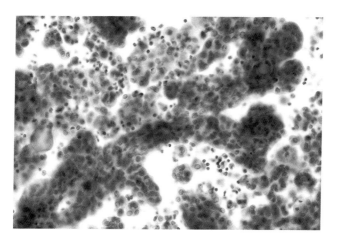

Fig. 4.12. *Malignant mesothelioma.* Hypercellular smear displaying the most characteristic architectural pattern of malignant mesothelioma, that is, a branching papillary-like configuration. Most metastases to the SCF will not display such a prominent papillary branching (with the exception of some gynecologic tract neoplasms) (Papanicolaou, low power).

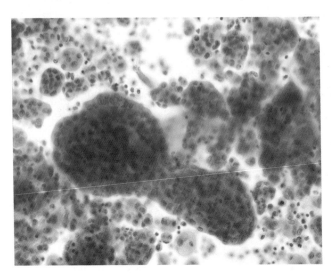

FIG. 4.13. *Malignant mesothelioma.* Small and large cellular fragments comprised of high N/C ratio cells are seen. The branching architecture is apparent as well as occasional single malignant cells in the smear background. The so-called one-cell pattern strongly supports a neoplastic process over a reactive hyperplasia of mesothelial cells (Papanicolaou, high power).

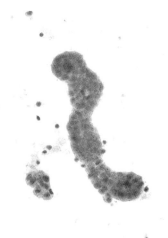

FIG. 4.14. *Malignant mesothelioma.* In this particular case, only rare malignant cells were observed. However, the neoplastic cells displayed a beautiful papillary-like architecture. These cellular fragments often display palisading of the peripherally placed cuboidal cells (Papanicolaou, high power).

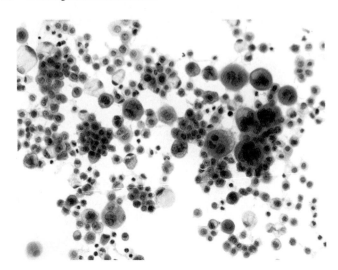

FIG. 4.15. *Malignant mesothelioma*. In this case of a pleural effusion, despite the two-cell population, the malignant nature of the cells is quite apparent. Cells are pleomorphic with frequent multinucleation, high N/C ratios, and nuclear hyperchromasia. Abundant benign mesothelial cells and few macrophages are also present (Papanicolaou, low power).

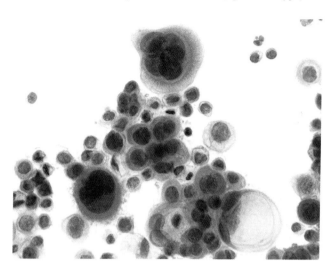

FIG. 4.16. *Malignant mesothelioma.* This is a beautiful illustration of diagnostic cellular findings in mesothelioma. The malignant cells show multinucleation with pleomorphic and enlarged nuclei and a distinct two-tone cytoplasmic texture. Also seen are cytoplasmic processes or the so-called whiskers (Papanicolaou, high power).

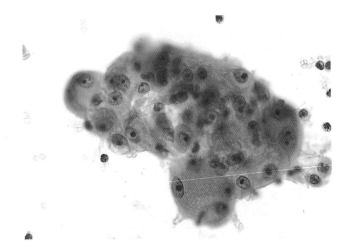

FIG. 4.17. *Malignant mesothelioma.* The presence of a single macronu-cleolus is an extremely helpful finding for the diagnosis of mesothelioma as opposed to reactive mesothelial hyperplasia. Metastatic adenocarcino-mas also display macronucleoli and therefore are the closest differential in this case. Also observed is a fine cytoplasmic vacuolization and well-defined cytoplasmic borders (Papanicolaou, high power).

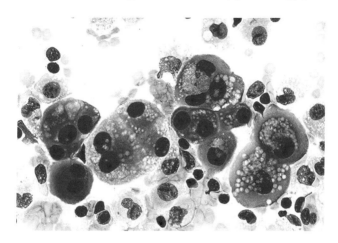

FIG. 4.18. *Malignant mesothelioma.* On Diff-Quik staining, the cytoplasmic vacuolization is often enhanced. These vacuoles are considered to represent intracytoplasmic lipid and can be stained with Oil Red O stain. A two-tone appearance of the cytoplasm is also seen as well as the characteristic binucleation and macronucleoli (Diff-Quik, high power).

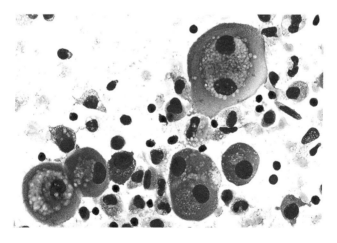

FIG. 4.19. *Malignant mesothelioma.* This is another illustration of binucleation, two-tone cytoplasmic texture, and macronucleoli. These characteristics are diagnostic of mesothelioma and are rarely observed in metastatic cancers (Diff-Quik, high power).

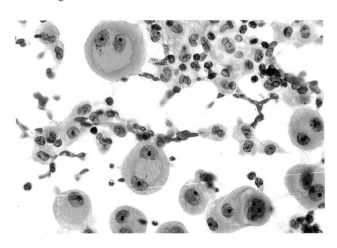

FIG. 4.20. *Malignant mesothelioma.* Singly placed malignant cells illustrating the diagnostic features of mesothelioma, that is, binucleation, two-tone cytoplasmic texture, centrally placed fine cytoplasmic vacuoles, and large nuclei containing macronucleoli (Papanicolaou, high power).

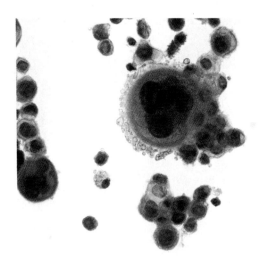

FIG. 4.21. *Malignant mesothelioma.* Higher magnification shows a multinucleated malignant cell with two-tone cytoplasm and characteristic cytoplasmic processes on the cell surface occasionally referred to as "cytoplasmic whiskers" or a "lacy" or "brush" border. This cytologic feature is rarely observed in metastatic carcinomas (Papanicolaou, high power).

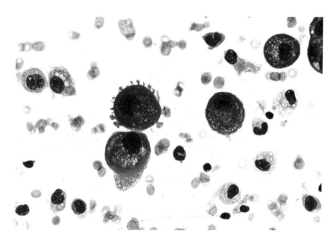

FIG. 4.22. *Malignant mesothelioma.* Another illustration of cytoplasmic whiskers in malignant cells is seen. Notice the centrally placed cytoplasmic microvacuoles and nuclei with macronucleoli. The presence of the cytoplasmic processes is often accentuated in smears stained with ultrafast Papanicolaou stain (not used here) when they are observed in the so-called retraction halos which surround individual malignant cells (Diff-Quik, high power).

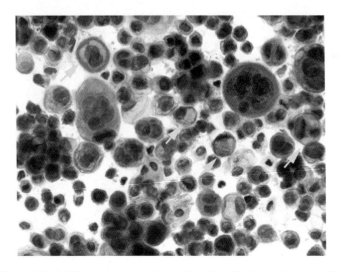

FIG. 4.23. *Malignant mesothelioma.* Occasionally, the malignant cells may contain pale yellow amorphous cytoplasmic substance (*arrows*). This substance likely represents accumulation of glycogen in these cells. This should not be confused with thick mucin of a metastatic adenocarcinoma (Papanicolaou, high power).

Malignant Mesothelioma – Other Cytomorphologic Features

- Fragments have irregularity of the outer contours – "scalloping" or "hob-nailed" look
- Centrally placed nuclei
- "Two-tone" cytoplasm (denser)
- Bi/multinucleation
- Fine cytoplasmic vacuoles
- Cytoplasmic processes

Malignant Mesothelioma (Epithelioid type) – Differential Diagnosis

- *Reactive mesothelial proliferation*
  - Lack of malignant cytologic features and tissue fragments
  - Florid mesothelial hyperplasia may be extremely difficult to differentiate from a well-differentiated mesothelioma

- *Metastatic neoplasms*
  - Adenocarcinoma
    - Both well- and poorly differentiated adenocarcinomas have features in common with mesothelioma
    - Definitive evidence of glandular differentiation may be extremely helpful
      - Acinus formation
      - Secretory vacuoles
      - Special stains (i.e., mucin and immunoperoxidase stains)

- *Other tumors*
  - (Anaplastic large-cell lymphoma, malignant melanoma, rhabdomyosarcoma) can be differentiated by identification of their specific cellular product or antigenic properties by employing special stains or other ancillary techniques

Malignant Mesothelioma vs. Adenocarcinoma

Epithelioid mesothelioma can be extremely difficult to differentiate from adenocarcinomas in SCF. Mucin stains (mucicarmine, periodic acid-Schiff [PAS] with diastase digestion, Alcian Blue or colloidal iron with hyaluronidase digestion) may help, but most laboratories are now performing immunostaining over enzyme cytochemistry.

Immunoperoxidase stains (mCEA, LeuM1, Ber-EP4, calretinin, CK 5/6, WT-1, and D2-40) may help in differential diagnosis. Determination of mucin in tumor cells and/or positive staining for mCEA, LeuM1, or Ber-EP4 indicates the epithelial origin of the tumor. These stains are negative in malignant mesothelioma as well as in reactive mesothelial cells, both of which stain with calretinin and markers of mesothelial differentiation (CK 5/6, WT-1, and D2-40). Cytokeratins AE1/AE3 are positive in both mesothelioma and adenocarcinoma and have no value in this regard. High-molecular-weight cytokeratins have been reported to be positive in mesothelioma but negative in adenocarcinoma. EMA stains both mesothelioma and adenocarcinoma; however, it often depicts a membranous or peripheral cytoplasmic accentuation in mesothelioma compared to metastatic adenocarcinoma.

Types of Mucins and Staining Results (Figs. 4.24 and 4.25)

- Mesothelioma – acid (mesenchymal) mucin hyaluronic acid
- Adenocarcinoma – neutral (epithelial) mucin
  - Mesothelioma – stains with PAS and Alcian Blue (but not with PAS-diastase or Alcian Blue-hyaluronic acid)
  - Adenocarcinoma – stains with all three, that is, mucicarmine, PAS (with and without diastase), and Alcian Blue (with and without hyaluronic acid)

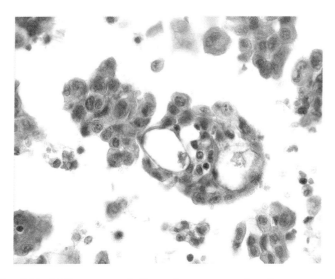

FIG. 4.24. *Malignant mesothelioma.* One way to confirm the presence of acidic mucin in mesothelioma cells is to perform Alcian Blue stain with and without hyaluronidase digestion. In this photomicrograph of a cell block section, the Alcian Blue stain is strongly positive in the intracytoplasmic vacuoles (high power).

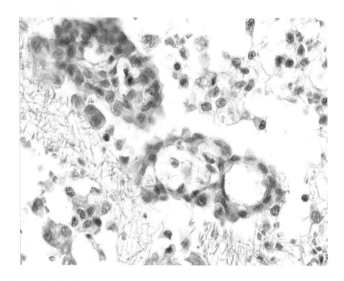

FIG. 4.25. *Malignant mesothelioma.* Same case as Fig. 4.24 is illustrated. In this case, Alcian Blue was done with hyaluronidase digestion resulting in a negative staining. This distinguishes a mesothelioma from a meta-static adenocarcinoma (the latter contains epithelial mucin and would not be affected by hyaluronidase digestion) (high power).

Disadvantages of Performing Special Cytochemical Stains

- Time-consuming to perform and interpret
- Offers no real advantage over immunoperoxidase labeling (except for the cost)
- Mucicarmine may show focal false positivity in ~10% of mesotheliomas
- Colloidal iron is a carcinogen and requires special handling

Mesothelioma vs. Adenocarcinoma – Immunoperoxidase Markers (Figs. 4.26, 4.27, 4.28, 4.29 and 4.30)

- Cytoskeletal proteins
- Cell surface glycoproteins
- Oncoplacental antigens
- Myelomonocytic antigens
- Intracellular calcium-binding proteins
- Cadherins
- Others

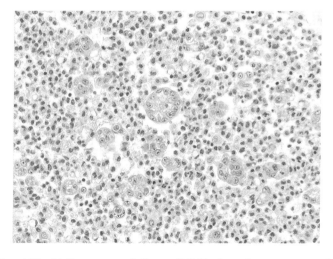

FIG. 4.26. *Malignant mesothelioma.* Cell block sections are extremely valuable in the workup of suspected cases of mesothelioma by providing additional cytomorphologic details as well as excellent material for further ancillary studies. As can be seen in this case, the three-dimensional balls of cells would raise the possibility of an adenocarcinoma (H & E, low power).

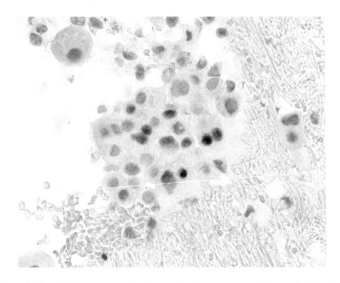

Fig. 4.27. *Malignant mesothelioma.* An immunoperoxidase stain for p53 displays strong nuclear reactivity helping to differentiate these cells from benign reactive mesothelial proliferation. p53 has excellent specificity for a cancer diagnosis but suffers from a comparatively low sensitivity (high power).

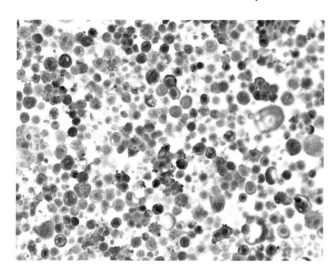

F<small>IG</small>. 4.28. *Malignant mesothelioma.* A calretinin immunostain is strongly and diffusely positive in the cytoplasm as well as nuclei of the malignant cells. A positive staining establishes a mesothelial differentiation in the cells but will not distinguish a benign from a malignant mesothelial process (low power).

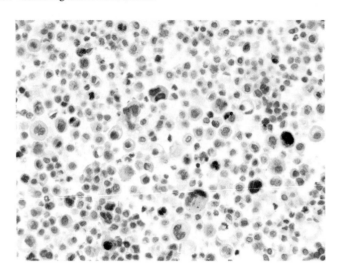

FIG. 4.29. *Malignant mesothelioma.* Another positive immunomarker helpful in establishing the diagnosis of mesothelioma when malignant cells are encountered is WT-1, which stains the nuclei. However, WT-1 stain is also positive in ovarian serous carcinomas and should be carefully interpreted in patients with history of ovarian cancer (low power).

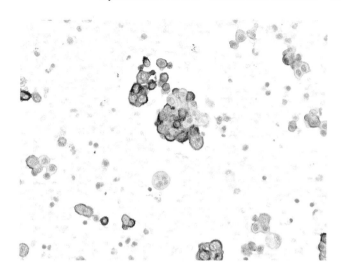

F<small>IG</small>. 4.30. *Malignant mesothelioma.* CK 5/6 is another useful marker to confirm mesothelial differentiation in malignant cells, as seen in this case with strong cytoplasmic membranous staining. When confirming the diagnosis of a mesothelioma, at least two of the three immunomarkers used should be positive (high power).

The following tables give salient positives and negatives of each immunomarker used:

Cytoskeletal Proteins – Intermediate Filaments

- Cytokeratins
- Vimentin

Cytokeratins, Vimentin – Diagnostic Utility

- CK (AE1/AE3, CAM5.2)
  - Almost all mesotheliomas and adenocarcinomas are positive
- Vimentin
  - Mesothelioma (epithelial) – scant or undetectable reaction
  - Adenocarcinoma – seldom (lung) to 50% positivity
    - Very confusing profile of limited value

Cell Surface Glycoproteins

- Epithelial membrane antigen (EMA)
- B72.3
- Ber-EP4
- Others (HEA-125, MOC-31, 44-3A6, and BG antigens)

Epithelial Membrane Antigen (EMA)

- Polymorphic epithelial mucin
- Mesothelioma – 5–42%
- Adenocarcinoma – 50–100%
- Membranous/spiky staining pattern in mesothelioma, focal staining in benign mesothelium
- Limited practical value

Monoclonal Antibody B72.3

- Mouse monoclonal AB, generated using human breast cancer cells
- Recognizes tumor-associated glycoprotein (TAG-72)
- Mesothelioma – 2–5% (weak)
- Adenocarcinoma – 80% (lung)

Monoclonal Antibody Ber-EP4

- Monoclonal antibody generated using MDF-7 breast carcinoma cell line
- Recognizes two glycopeptides on normal epithelium and carcinoma
- Mesothelioma – 0–26% (focal)
- Adenocarcinoma – 92%

Oncoplacental Antigens

- Carcinoembryonic antigen (CEA)
- Placental antigen (PLAP)

Carcinoembryonic Antigen (CEA)

- Oldest and most widely used antibody in the diagnosis of adenocarcinoma vs. mesothelioma
- Mesothelioma – 15–45% with pCEA
- Adenocarcinoma – 85–95% (lung)
- Papillary serous carcinoma – 16%

Placental Alkaline Phosphatase (PLAP)

- Mesothelioma – 15%
- Adenocarcinoma (lung) – 19–67%
- Papillary serous carcinoma – 24–63%

Myelomonocytic Antigens

- LeuM1 (CD15)
- LN2 (CD74)

LeuM1 (CD15)

- Monoclonal antibody, recognizes glycolipid sugar sequence
- Reed-Sternberg cell marker
- Mesothelioma – 0–32%
- Adenocarcinoma – 42–94%
- Highly useful and specific marker (although comparatively less sensitive)

Intracytoplasmic Ca++– Binding Proteins

- Calretinin
- S-100 protein

Calretinin

- 29-kDa Ca++-binding protein
- Expressed by neurons, gonads, adipose tissue, kidney, sweat glands, thymus, and mesothelium
- Mesothelioma – 42–100%
- Adenocarcinoma (lung) – 6–20% (focal)
- Small-cell carcinoma – 49%
- Most useful positive marker for mesothelium

S-100 protein

- Mesothelioma – 0%
- Adenocarcinoma (lung) – 17%
- Papillary serous carcinoma – 31%
- Limited diagnostic value

Combined E-Cadherin and Calretinin Immunostaining

• *E-cadherin* – Ca-dependent CAM, specific for epithelia		
	E-cadherin	*Calretinin*
Reactive mesothelium	0%	100%
Mesothelioma	100%	100%
Adenocarcinoma	86.5%	0%
Interpretation		
Reactive mesothelium	–	+
Mesothelioma	+	+
Adenocarcinoma	+	–
Kitazume et al., Cancer Cytopathol, 2000		

Other Mesothelioma Markers

CK 5/6

- Epithelioid mesothelioma – 83%
- Sarcomatoid mesothelioma – 26%
- Adenocarcinoma: pancreatic – 35%, lung – 8–65%

D2-40

- Monoclonal antibody directed against human podoplanin
- Transmembrane mucoprotein expressed in lymphatic endothelial cells
- Positive in lymphovascular neoplasms (lymphangioma, Kaposi's sarcoma, hemangioendothelioma), nonvascular neoplasms (epithelioid mesothelioma, seminoma, hemangioblastoma, primary adrenal cortical tumors, schwannoma, skin adnexal tumors)
- D2-40 immunostains 66% of the epithelioid and 30% of the sarcomatoid mesotheliomas (compared to calretinin which stains 91% of epithelioid and 57% of sarcomatoid mesotheliomas)
- Strong membranous staining for epithelioid mesothelioma
- Combination of calretinin and D2-40 improves diagnostic accuracy for sarcomatoid mesothelioma
- Lung adenocarcinoma (36%) may show a focal weak to moderate cytoplasmic only expression

WT-1

- Transcription factor, the gene product of Wilms' tumor 1
- As a tumor suppressor gene
- WT-1 protein is normally expressed in the developing genitourinary tract, heart, spleen, and adrenal glands and is crucial for their development

- Ninety-two percent of ovarian serous carcinomas and 80% of peritoneal serous carcinomas express WT-1
- Useful in distinguishing ovarian serous carcinoma from uterine serous carcinoma (characteristically negative)
- Mesothelioma – 74%, lung adenocarcinoma – 0%

Role of CK 7 and CK 20

- Limited role
- Mesothelioma is CK 7+, CK 20–
- Most common metastases to SCF (breast, lung, and ovary) are also CK 7+, CK 20–

Mesothelioma vs. Adenocarcinoma – Johns Hopkins Cytopathology Lab Immunopanel

Stain	Mesothelioma	Adenocarcinoma
mCEA	3%	85–95%
Ber-EP4	0–26%	92%
LeuM1	0–32%	42–94%
Calretinin	65–100%	6–20% (focal, weak)
CK 5/6	83%	8–65%
WT-1	78%	0%
D2-40	66%	36% (focal, weak)

Cytogenetic Analysis of Effusions from Malignant Mesothelioma

- Distinguish malignant from reactive mesothelial cells
- Direct metaphase harvests and short-term cultures may be performed on fresh fluid
- Clonal cytogenetic aberrations indicative of malignancy – Del(1p), Del(3p), and Del(22q)

FISH Analysis of Effusions from Malignant Mesothelioma

- FISH with centromeric chromosome 7 and 9 probes
- Destained Diff-Quik-stained smears
- Chromosome 7
  - Polysomy (88%)
  - Trisomy (77%)
  - Tetrasomy (29%)

- Chromosome 9
  - Polysomy (69%)
  - Trisomy (62%)

Selected Reading

Bailey ME, Brown RW, Mody DR, Cagle P, Ramzy I. Ber-EP4 for differentiating adenocarcinoma from reactive and neoplastic mesothelial cells in serous effusions. Comparison with carcinoembryonic antigen, B72.3 and Leu-M1. Acta Cytol. 1996;40(6):1212–6.

Bedrossian CW. Diagnostic problems in serous effusions. Diagn Cytopathol. 1998;19(2):131–7.

Davidson B. The diagnostic and molecular characteristics of malignant mesothelioma and ovarian/peritoneal serous carcinoma. Cytopathology. 2011;22(1):5–21. Epub 2010 Nov 30.

DiBonito L, Falconieri G, Colautti I, Bonifacio Gori D, Dudine S, Giarelli L. Cytopathology of malignant mesothelioma: a study of its patterns and histological bases. Diagn Cytopathol. 1993;9(1):25–31.

Granados R, Cibas ES, Fletcher JA. Cytogenetic analysis of effusions from malignant mesothelioma. A diagnostic adjunct to cytology. Acta Cytol. 1994;38(5):711–7.

Kho-Duffin J, Tao LC, Cramer H, Catellier MJ, Irons D, Ng P. Cytologic diagnosis of malignant mesothelioma, with particular emphasis on the epithelial noncohesive cell type. Diagn Cytopathol. 1999;20(2):57–62.

Lee JS, Nam JH, Lee MC, Park CS, Juhng SW. Immunohistochemical panel for distinguishing between carcinoma and reactive mesothelial cells in serious effusions. Acta Cytol. 1996;40(4):631–6.

Lozano MD, Panizo A, Toledo GR, Sola JJ, Pardo-Mindán J. Immunocytochemistry in the differential diagnosis of serous effusions: a comparative evaluation of eight monoclonal antibodies in Papanicolaou stained smears. Cancer. 2001;93(1):68–72.

Motoyama T, Watanabe T, Okazaki E, Tanaka N, Watanabe H. Immuno-histochemical properties of malignant mesothelioma cells in histologic and cytologic specimens. Acta Cytol. 1995;39(2):164–70.

Naylor B. The exfoliative cytology of diffuse malignant mesothelioma. J Pathol Bacteriol. 1963;86:293–8.

Raja S, Murthy SC, Mason DP. Malignant pleural mesothelioma. Curr Oncol Rep. 2011;13:259–64.

Rakha EA, Patil S, Abdulla K, Abdulkader M, Chaudry Z, Soomro IN. The sensitivity of cytologic evaluation of pleural fluid in the diagnosis of malignant mesothelioma. Diagn Cytopathol. 2010;38(12):874–9.

Stevens MW, Leong AS, Fazzalari NL, Dowling KD, Henderson DW. Cytopathology of malignant mesothelioma: a stepwise logistic regression analysis. Diagn Cytopathol. 1992;8(4):333–41.

5
Metastatic Cancers

Although a variety of nonneoplastic entities (inflammatory processes and infectious) can be adequately diagnosed on cytologic
analysis of serous cavity fluids (SCFs), the most common clinical reason is to exclude a malignant process. Malignant mesothelioma is the most common primary tumor of the serosal membrane;
however, a metastatic cancer (more specifically adenocarcinoma)
is by far the most frequently encountered malignant tumor in SCFs.
Malignant cells, when observed in SCF, impart poor prognostic significance to an oncologic patient by defining a higher clinical stage.
Frequency analysis showed the incidence of carcinoma of the lung
to be the most common cause of malignant effusion (Hsu).

Adenocarcinoma (Figs. 5.1, 5.2, 5.3, 5.4, 5.5, 5.6, 5.7, 5.8, 5.9, 5.10, 5.11, 5.12, 5.13, 5.14, 5.15, 5.16, 5.17, 5.18, 5.19, 5.20, 5.21, 5.22, 5.23 and 5.24)

- Most common metastases to the serosa
- Lung, breast, and ovary – most common primaries

(continued)

S.Z. Ali and E.S. Cibas, *Serous Cavity Fluid and Cerebrospinal Fluid Cytopathology*, Essentials in Cytopathology 10, DOI 10.1007/ 978-1-4614-1776-7_5,
© Springer Science+Business Media, LLC 2012

- Cytologic patterns
  - Predominantly tissue fragments
  - Lobular breast carcinoma and some poorly differentiated carcinomas may have predominantly single cells
  - Ductal breast carcinoma may show three-dimensional spheres or "cannon balls" and occasionally single bland-appearing cells "mesothelial pattern"
  - Acinus formation
  - Papillary architecture
  - Secretory vacuoles
  - Mucin stains and immunochemistry can be helpful in difficult cases

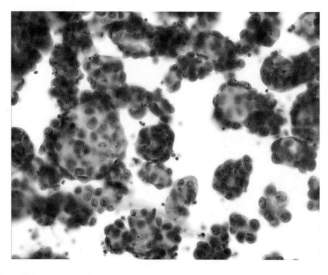

Fig. 5.1. *Lung adenocarcinoma. Pleural effusion.* Numerous three-dimensional fragments of malignant cells are seen. Note the hollowness of the central portion of these cellular fragments representing a true acinus (or lumen) formation. In contrast, similar cellular fragments in mesothelioma would contain a *pale green* submesothelial matrix tissue (Papanicolaou, low power).

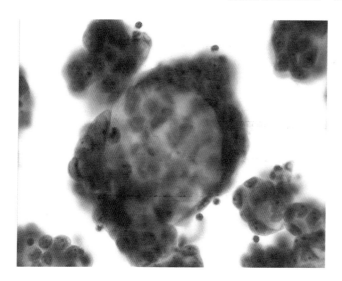

FIG. 5.2. *Lung adenocarcinoma. Pleural effusion.* Higher magnification illustrates the sharply punched out lumen in the center of a cellular fragment surrounded by high N/C ratio carcinoma cells with prominent nucleoli (Papanicolaou, high power).

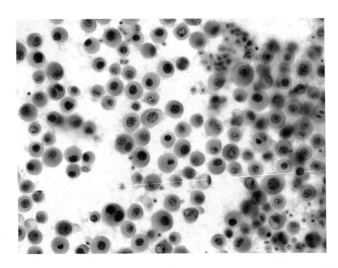

FIG. 5.3. *Lung adenocarcinoma. Pleural effusion.* In this patient with a long history of asbestos exposure, these cells strongly raise the possibility of a malignant mesothelioma. The predominant cytoarchitecture is that of single cells with *round* to *oval* nuclei and slightly opaque cytoplasm. Follow-up was consistent with involvement by a lung adenocarcinoma (Papanicolaou, low power).

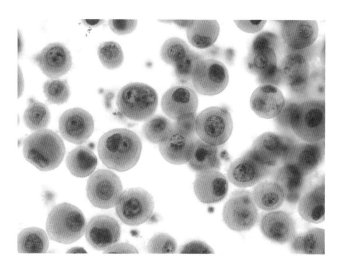

FIG. 5.4. *Lung adenocarcinoma. Pleural effusion.* Higher magnification also shows binucleation and prominent nucleoli. A malignant mesothelioma needs to be carefully excluded by a panel of immunostains in such cases (Papanicolaou, high power).

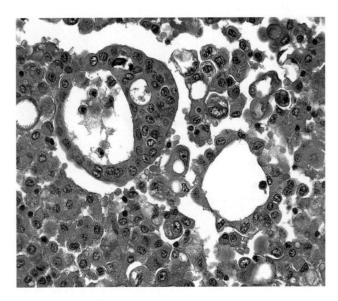

FIG. 5.5. *Lung adenocarcinoma. Pleural effusion.* A cell block section in the same case clearly supports the diagnosis of a metastatic carcinoma with smooth contoured outer borders of the glandular fragments and lumens containing mucin. Background contains numerous reactive mesothelial cells and histiocytes (H & E, high power).

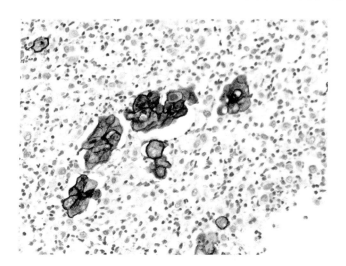

FIG. 5.6. *Lung adenocarcinoma. Pleural effusion.* A Ber-EP4 immunostain confirms the epithelial nature of the cells in this case consistent with the diagnosis of an adenocarcinoma. Note the negative background mesothelial cells and histiocytes. Ber-EP4 is one of the immunostains with the "cleanest" staining pattern in SCFs where a large number of histiocytes are often a problem causing "dirty" slide background staining (low power).

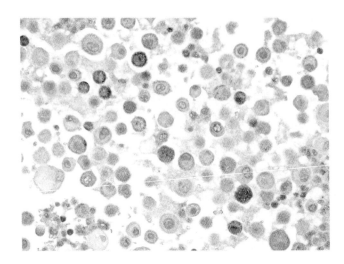

FIG. 5.7. *Lung adenocarcinoma. Pleural effusion.* A monoclonal CEA immunostain strongly decorates the singly dispersed adenocarcinoma cells in this case. An mCEA stain is usually quite specific for epithelial differentiation as opposed to polyclonal subtype of the marker (high power).

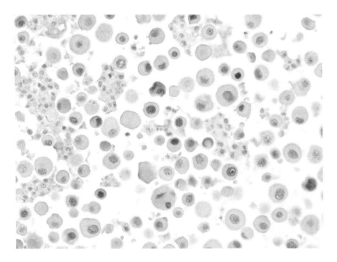

FIG. 5.8. *Lung adenocarcinoma. Pleural effusion.* A TTF-1 immunostain is beautifully positive in the neoplastic cell nuclei confirming the pulmonary origin of the adenocarcinoma (high power).

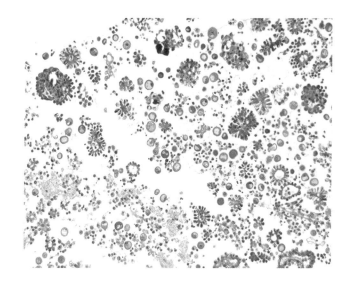

Fɪɢ. 5.9. *Micropapillary lung adenocarcinoma. Pleural fluid.* This uncommon variant of lung adenocarcinoma with an aggressive biological behavior illustrates a beautiful papillary architecture with occasional psammoma bodies (1 o'clock). This tumor frequently manifests at higher clinical stage with a poor prognosis and frequently metastasizes to the contralateral lung, mediastinal lymph nodes, bone, and adrenal glands, with high mortality (Papanicolaou, low power).

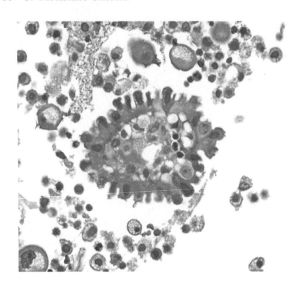

FIG. 5.10. *Micropapillary lung adenocarcinoma. Pleural fluid.* Higher magnification of the previous case shows a well-formed glandular fragment with characteristic hob-nailed nuclei protruding outward (reverse polarity). Nuclei show prominent nucleoli. Micropapillary growth patterns have been associated with an aggressive clinical course compared with traditional papillary adenocarcinoma and bronchioloalveolar carcinoma (Papanicolaou, high power).

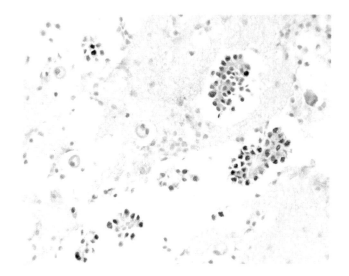

FIG. 5.11. *Micropapillary lung carcinoma. Pleural fluid.* A positive TTF-1 immunostain confirms the pulmonary origin of the carcinoma in this case. Studies have shown a much higher expression of K-ras, *EGFR*, and BRAF mutations in adenocarcinomas of lung with a dominant micropapillary growth pattern compared with conventional adenocarcinoma (Papanicolaou, low power).

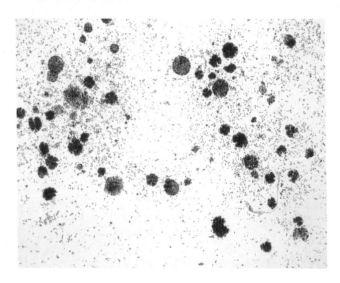

FIG. 5.12. *Breast ductal carcinoma. Pleural effusion.* Although any metastatic adenocarcinoma in SCF can create three-dimensional cellular balls, this phenomenon is best illustrated in cases of metastatic breast ductal carcinoma. These cellular fragments are also referred to as "proliferation spheres" or "cannon balls" (Papanicolaou, low power).

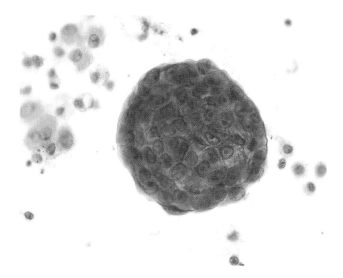

FIG. 5.13. *Breast ductal carcinoma. Pleural effusion.* A three-dimensional ball of malignant epithelial cells displaying the characteristic smooth outer border created by fusion of the cytoplasmic membranes of the adjacent cells. This phenomenon is highly characteristic of adenocarcinomas in SCF and is often referred to as "the community border." This is in sharp contrast to the irregular outer border of mesothelioma cells, the latter due to hob nailing of the markedly enlarged nuclei. Each malignant cell in mesothelioma fragment would retain its own cytoplasmic border (Papanicolaou, high power).

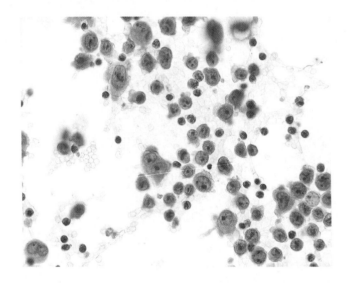

FIG. 5.14. *Breast ductal carcinoma. Pleural effusion.* Another phenotypic appearance of breast ductal carcinoma is the so-called single cell mesothelial pattern. The malignant cells are seen singly dispersed with large eccentrically placed nuclei with prominent nucleoli. This feature is in sharp contrast to the mostly centrally placed nuclei of mesothelioma cells, which are often binucleated or multinucleated as well (Papanicolaou, high power).

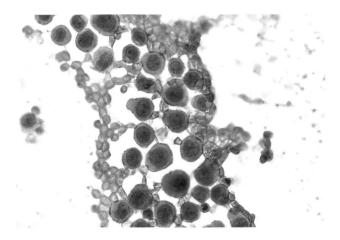

FIG. 5.15. *Breast ductal carcinoma. Pleural effusion.* Another illustration of the so-called mesothelial pattern of the ductal carcinoma cells in SCF is pictured. Notice the cytoplasmic opacity in these cells further creating diagnostic confusion with benign mesothelial cells or uncommonly with mesothelioma. The nuclei show markedly convoluted and irregular outlines (Papanicolaou, high power).

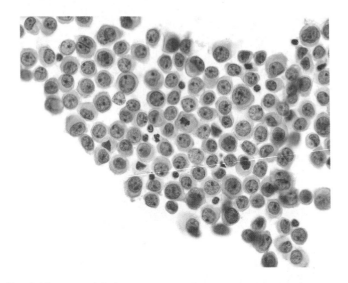

FIG. 5.16. *Breast lobular carcinoma. Pleural effusion.* A notoriously difficult diagnosis in SCF is that of metastatic lobular breast carcinoma. This is due to the fact that the malignant cells are predominantly dispersed, singly placed, and due to their relatively smaller size and high N/C ratios may resemble contaminating lymphocytes. However, the presence of mitoses and occasional nucleoli will help in proper identification especially when a substantial amount of malignant cells are present (as in this case) (Papanicolaou, high power).

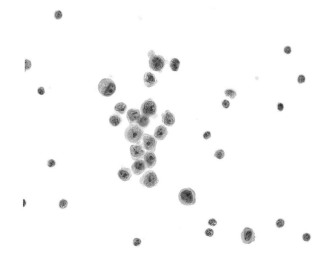

FIG. 5.17. *Breast lobular carcinoma. Pleural effusion.* Depicted is another example which displays high N/C ratio smaller cells with prominent nucleoli. In cases with heavy mesothelial and inflammatory cell contamination, malignant lobular carcinoma cells are very hard to appreciate and immunostains need to be performed if there is a history of a breast primary (Papanicolaou, high power).

FIG. 5.18. *Breast lobular carcinoma. Pleural effusion.* Although Indian-filing is a histologic feature of breast lobular carcinoma, occasional cases of SCF may illustrate similar cytoarchitecture, as seen in this case. Notice the lymphocyte-like nature of the carcinoma cells (Papanicolaou, high power).

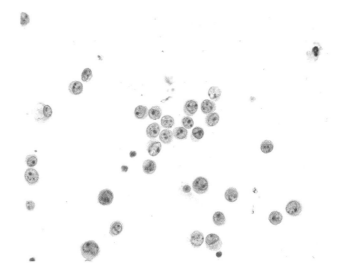

FIG. 5.19. *Gastric adenocarcinoma. Peritoneal fluid.* Another type of carcinoma where the malignant cells display the phenotypic appearance similar to a breast lobular carcinoma is that of a gastric primary. These high N/C ratio cells should be carefully differentiated from a malignant lymphomatous process by immunostaining. In this case, the patient had a known history of a "linitis plastica–type" stomach cancer (Papanicolaou, high power).

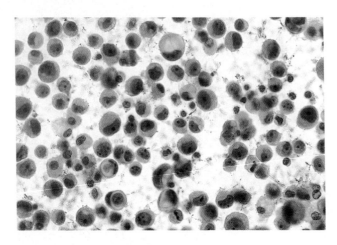

FIG. 5.20. *Gastric signet-ring adenocarcinoma. Ascitic fluid.* Another common phenotypic appearance of gastric cancer is a signet-ring-type cytomorphology. As seen here, the malignant cells display large cytoplasmic vacuoles containing mucin with eccentrically placed nuclei and macronucleoli. These cells need to be differentiated from pseudo signet-ring cells commonly observed in cases of hepatic cirrhosis (Papanicolaou, high power).

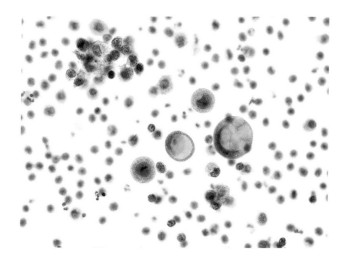

F<small>IG</small>. 5.21. *Gastric signet-ring adenocarcinoma. Peritoneal fluid.* Higher magnification of another case beautifully illustrates large cytoplasmic vacuoles indenting the nuclei and pushing them to the edge of the cell (Papanicolaou, high power).

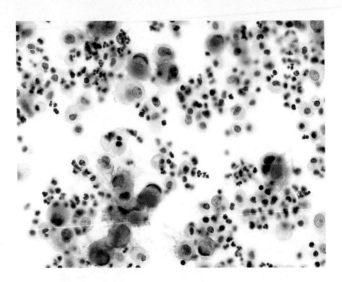

FIG. 5.22. *Gastric signet-ring adenocarcinoma. Peritoneal fluid.* The easiest way to confirm the presence of intracytoplasmic mucin is to perform a mucicarmine stain. In this smear, intracytoplasmic mucin is highlighted by a strong and crisp orange-red staining (high power).

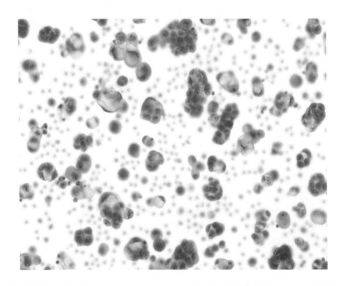

FIG. 5.23. *Ovarian serous carcinoma. Ascitic fluid.* A large population of malignant cells forming three-dimensional balls of varying sizes is seen. Intracytoplasmic vacuoles are also visible in most of the fragments (Papanicolaou, low power).

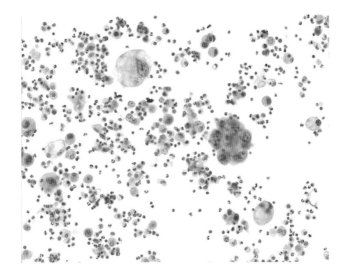

FIG. 5.24. *Ovarian serous carcinoma. Ascitic fluid.* The high-grade nature of malignant cells is quite obvious in this case due to extensive pleomorphism. The high N/C ratio cells contain macronucleoli, and the background shows inflammatory necrosis (Papanicolaou, low power).

Adenocarcinoma – Differential Diagnosis

- Malignant mesothelioma
- Anaplastic large-cell lymphoma (Ki-1 positive)
- Anaplastic myeloma
- Malignant melanoma
- Metastatic tumors with "epithelioid" morphology

Squamous Cell Carcinoma
(Figs. 5.25, 5.26 and 5.27)

- Rarely exfoliates in effusions (less than 1% of all effusions)
- Usually discloses evidence of squamous differentiation/
  keratinization and apparent malignant features

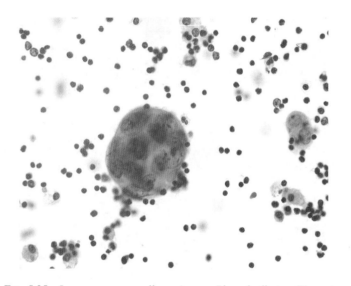

FIG. 5.25. *Lung squamous cell carcinoma. Pleural effusion.* The cytologic features strongly suggest an adenocarcinoma in this case due to the
presence of a tight ball of malignant epithelial cells. Note the smooth outer
edge of the cellular fragment. However, this patient has an advanced stage
lung squamous cell carcinoma. Due to the rarity of metastasis to SCFs and
in the absence of obvious keratinization, squamous cell carcinomas are
often hard to diagnose in effusion specimens (Papanicolaou, high power).

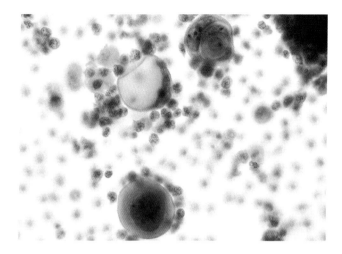

FIG. 5.26. *Lung squamous cell carcinoma. Pleural effusion.* A rare metastasis to SCF, squamous cell carcinomas are easily diagnosable when orangeophilic cytoplasmic keratinization is evident. However, as seen in this case, the differential diagnosis will also involve an adenocarcinoma due to the cells containing cytoplasmic vacuoles. The cells at 1 o'clock display the cell-in-cell appearance or the so-called cell cannibalism. This phenomenon can be seen in mesotheliomas as well. The cell at 6 o'clock displays a distinct cytoplasmic opacity likely reflecting keratinization (Papanicolaou, high power).

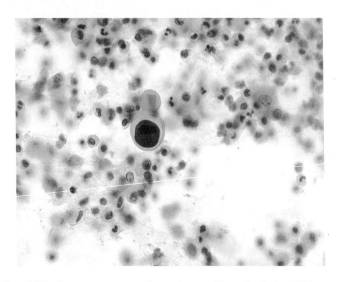

Fig. 5.27. *Lung squamous cell carcinoma. Pleural effusion.* This case clearly displays a malignant keratinized squamous cell with the so-called Halloween *orange color* of the cytoplasm. Rarely, squamous cell metaplasia may occur in serosal lining resulting in occasional mature-appearing cells in the effusions (Papanicolaou, high power).

Small-Cell Carcinoma (Figs. 5.28, 5.29, 5.30, 5.31, 5.32, 5.33 and 5.34)

- Uncommon in pleural effusions
- Usually seen as small tissue fragments
- Cellular (cytoplasm to nuclear) molding, formation of columns (vertebra-like), and concentric round (onion-skin-like) formations
- Cellular characteristics
  - High N/C ratio and lack of conspicuous nucleoli
  - Finely granular chromatin
  - Tight nuclear molding, or less commonly, single lymphocyte-like dispersed nuclei
  - Karyorrhexis and mitoses

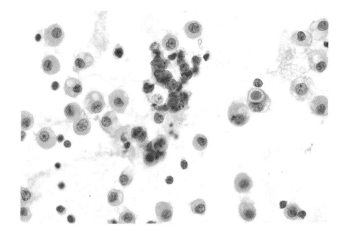

FIG. 5.28. *Lung small-cell carcinoma. Pericardial effusion.* Another uncommon metastasis to SCF is a small-cell carcinoma. These cases can be extremely hard to diagnose when a small population of malignant cells is present, often overshadowed and diluted by abundant background mesothelial cells and histiocytes. In this case the malignant cells are seen tightly molded against each other displaying hyperchromatic nuclei (Papanicolaou, high power).

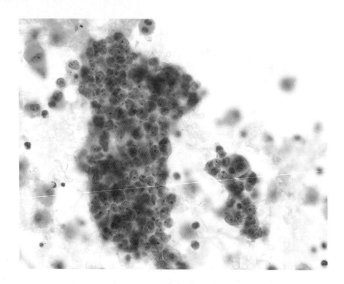

FIG. 5.29. *Lung small-cell carcinoma. Pericardial effusion.* This is another example where a large volume of malignant cells was encountered. Diagnostic features are the relatively smaller cell size, high N/C ratios with most cells appearing as naked nuclei, nuclear hyperchromasia, and tight cell-to-cell molding (Papanicolaou, high power).

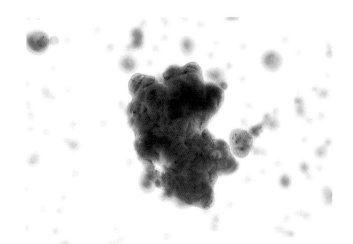

FIG. 5.30. *Lung, small-cell carcinoma. Pericardial effusion.* High magnification in a case beautifully illustrates hyperchromasia and tight nuclear molding of the adjacent cells. Also notice the lack of nucleoli in neoplastic cells with evenly distributed and finely granular chromatin (Papanicolaou, high power).

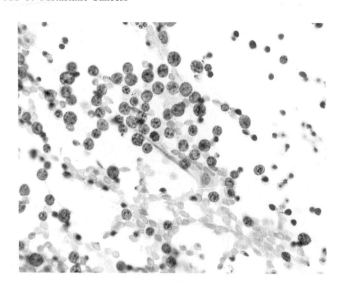

FIG. 5.31. *Lung small-cell carcinoma. Pericardial effusion.* This particular case was difficult to differentiate from malignant non-Hodgkin's lymphoma due to a single cell dispersed pattern. Confirmatory immunostains have to be performed before a definitive diagnosis is made in such cases (Papanicolaou, high power).

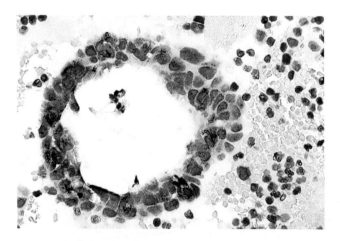

FIG. 5.32. *Lung small-cell carcinoma. Pericardial effusion.* Cell block section with a strong immunoreactivity with synaptophysin in a granular cytoplasmic pattern confirms the diagnosis in the above case (high power).

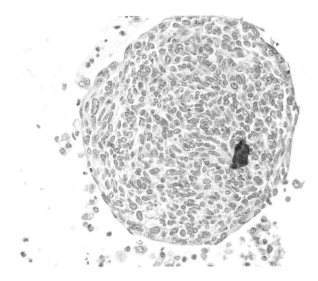

Fɪɢ. 5.33. *Lung small-cell carcinoma. Pleural effusion.* This cell block section from another case illustrates a morule-like architecture with small uniform round to oval malignant cells tightly wrapped around and forming a cellular ball. This unusual architecture is often observed in cell block sections of metastatic small-cell carcinomas (H & E, high power).

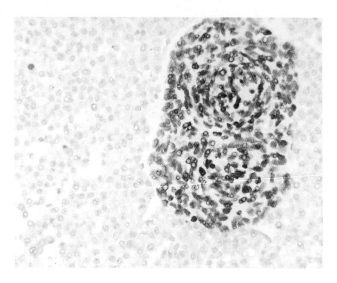

FIG. 5.34. *Lung small-cell carcinoma. Pleural effusion.* On immunostaining in the prior case, the malignant cell nuclei strongly stained with TTF-1 confirming the pulmonary origin of the primary site. It is worthwhile to remember that small-cell carcinomas from other body sites may also immunostain with TTF-1. Clinical and/or radiologic history of a lung mass is extremely helpful in such cases (high power).

Small-Cell Carcinoma – Differential Diagnosis

- Other "small blue cell" tumors
- Adenocarcinoma of breast, endometrium, and prostate
  - May form fragments with cellular molding but usually have prominent nucleoli and well-discernible cytoplasm

- Malignant NHL
  - Single discohesive cells

- Other small round tumors
  - Carcinoid and PanNET
  - Ewing's sarcoma/PNET

Miscellaneous Other Cancers (Figs. 5.26, 5.27, 5.28, 5.29, 5.30, 5.31, 5.32, 5.33, 5.34, 5.35, 5.36, 5.37, 5.38, 5.39, 5.40, 5.41, 5.42, 5.43, 5.44, 5.45, 5.46, 5.47, 5.48, 5.49, 5.50, 5.51, 5.52, 5.53, 5.54, 5.55, 5.56, 5.57, 5.58, 5.59 and 5.60)

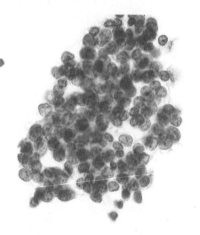

FIG. 5.35. *Merkel cell carcinoma. Pleural effusion.* The malignant cells have strong phenotypic resemblance to the previous cases of small-cell carcinoma. As a matter of fact, morphologic distinction between Merkel cell carcinoma of the skin and small-cell carcinoma from other body sites cannot be made, and confirmatory immunostains are always required. Malignant cells in this case display extreme hyperchromasia and an almost naked nuclear population (Papanicolaou, high power).

Malignant Melanoma

- Cytomorphologic features
  - Single cells and small tissue fragments
  - Epithelial and sarcomatous features
  - Large nuclei with macronucleoli
  - Intranuclear pseudo inclusions
  - Intracytoplasmic melanin pigment
  - Amelanotic melanoma may require immunostaining (Melan-A, HMB-45, and S-100 protein) to confirm the diagnosis

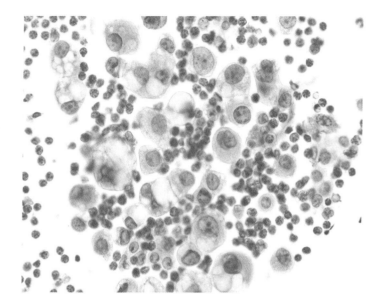

FIG. 5.36. *Renal cell carcinoma. Peritoneal effusion.* Depicted are significantly larger malignant cells with distinctly vacuolated cytoplasm (so-called soap bubble appearance) and macronucleoli. Renal cell carcinoma rarely metastasizes to SCF (Papanicolaou, high power).

Malignant Melanoma – Differential Diagnosis

- Variety of sarcomas may metastasize to the serosal surface
- Clinical history and ancillary studies (immunostaining, EM, and cytogenetics) may be needed to establish an accurate diagnosis

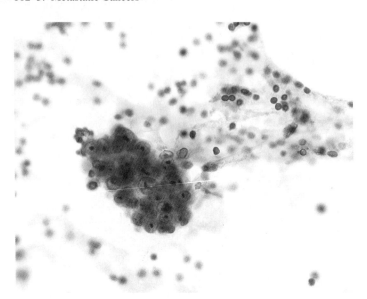

FIG. 5.37.   *Renal collecting duct carcinoma. Pleural effusion.* Neoplastic cells in this case have phenotypic resemblance to an adenocarcinoma with round to oval nuclei, vesicular chromatin, and macronucleoli. A previous history of a renal primary is extremely crucial to avoid misdiagnosis in this rare tumor (Papanicolaou, high power).

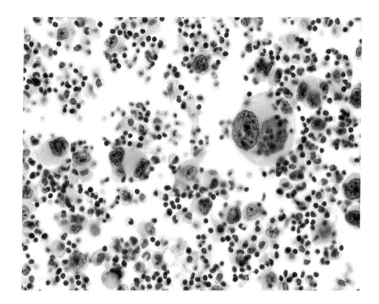

FIG. 5.38. *Urothelial carcinoma. Pleural effusion.* Pleomorphic malignant cells with enlarged hyperchromatic nuclei, single or multiple nucleoli, and opaque cytoplasm are seen in a single cell pattern. Once again, the previous history of a urinary tract malignancy is extremely important in this case where classic features of urothelial differentiation are missing (Papanicolaou, high power).

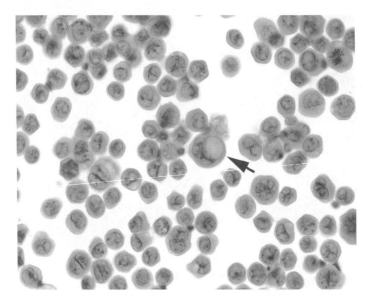

FIG. 5.39. *Signet-ring cell urothelial carcinoma. Peritoneal fluid.* This unusual case illustrates a rare variant of urothelial carcinoma. Notice the well-formed signet-ring cells (*arrow*). All cells in this field illustrating high N/C ratios and mitoses are consistent with metastases from the known urothelial primary in this patient (Papanicolaou, high power).

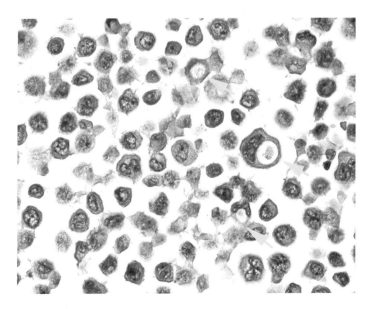

Fɪɢ. 5.40. *Signet-ring cell urothelial carcinoma. Peritoneal fluid.* Cell block section illustrates the signet-ring cell morphology and other malignant features of the neoplastic cells (H & E, high power).

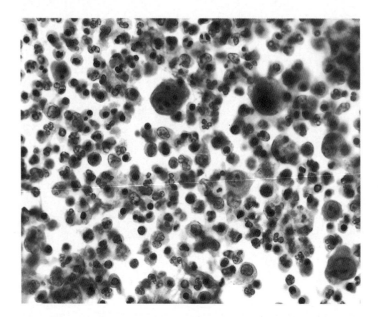

FIG. 5.41. *Anaplastic thyroid carcinoma. Pleural effusion.* Metastasis from a thyroid primary to SCF is rare. In this case of an advanced stage anaplastic carcinoma, the large cells seen here have obvious malignant features (pleomorphism, large nuclei with macronucleoli) and are seen in an inflamed background. A morphologic diagnosis without the known history and/or immunostaining would not have been possible in this case (Papanicolaou, high power).

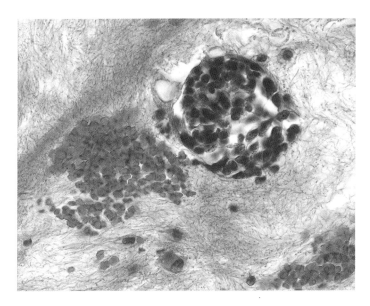

FIG. 5.42. *Glioblastoma multiforme (GBM). Pleural effusion.* Extracranial metastasis of primary brain tumors is exceedingly rare. In this unusual case of a metastatic small-cell GBM, the neoplastic cells are seen in this cell block section resembling a neuroendocrine carcinoma (H & E, high power).

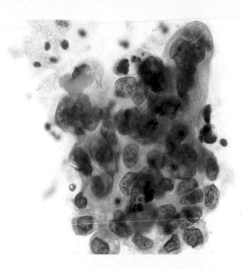

FIG. 5.43. *Choriocarcinoma. Ascitic fluid.* In this unusual case, the malignant cells are large and pleomorphic, often displaying multinucleation. History of a previous germ cell tumor is imperative to arrive at an accurate diagnosis. Additionally, immunostains have to be performed in such rare tumors to confirm the diagnosis (Papanicolaou, high power).

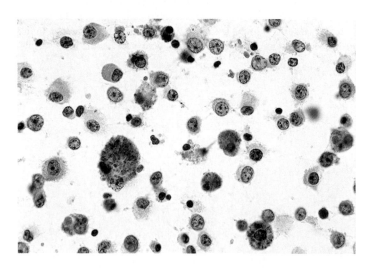

FIG. 5.44. *Malignant melanoma. Pleural effusion.* This SCF was grossly noticed to be dark brown in a patient with known history of melanoma. Cytomorphology is highlighted by abundant melanophages explaining the *dark color* of the effusion in this case. The background cells, some with macronucleoli, are the malignant melanoma cells. In cases like this, immunostains are often not needed (Papanicolaou, high power).

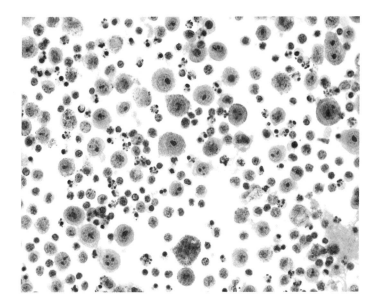

FIG. 5.45. *Malignant melanoma. Pleural effusion.* This case illustrates a much larger population of malignant cells with eccentric nuclei and macronucleoli. Additionally, numerous melanophages are present (Papanicolaou, low power).

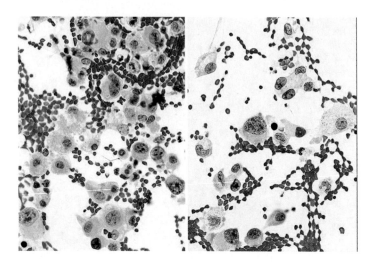

Fig. 5.46. *Malignant melanoma. Ascitic fluid.* Occasionally, one may encounter amelanotic tumors. In this case, the malignant cells appear pleomorphic with eccentric nuclei and binucleation. Confirmatory immunostains may be needed since no melanin is seen. Occasional cells have cytoplasmic characteristics of histiocytes (Papanicolaou, high power).

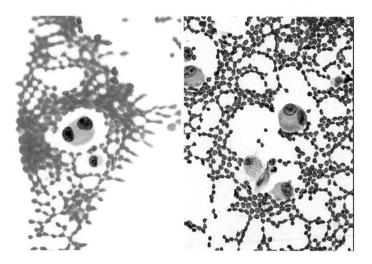

Fig. 5.47. *Malignant melanoma. Ascitic fluid.* These examples illustrate the characteristic binucleation of a metastatic melanoma. Also noticed are macronucleoli (Papanicolaou, high power).

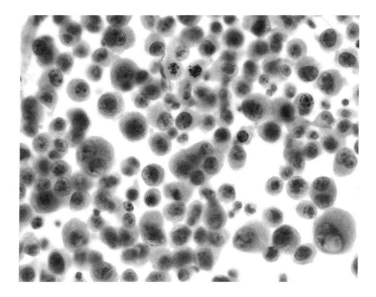

FIG. 5.48. *Malignant melanoma. Pleural effusion.* In this example of melanoma, the malignant cells have a prominent epithelioid morphology with eccentrically placed large nuclei and macronucleoli. Numerous mitotic figures are also evident. Confirmatory immunostains are needed (Papanicolaou, high power).

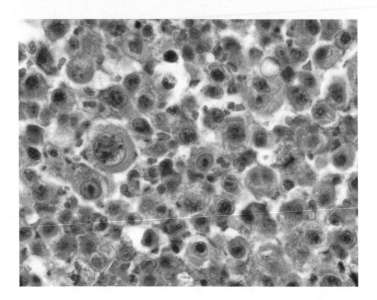

FIG. 5.49. *Malignant melanoma. Pleural effusion.* The malignant cells display extreme anisonucleosis with eccentrically placed nuclei, macronucleoli, and mitoses. Due to phenotypic resemblance with metastatic carcinoma in this cell block section, the diagnosis should be confirmed by a panel of immunostains (H & E, high power).

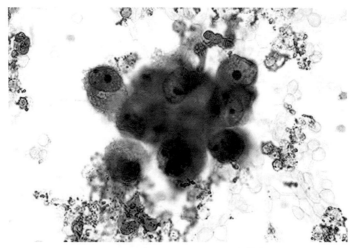

FIG. 5.50. *Epithelioid hemangioendothelioma. Pleural effusion.* Mesenchymal neoplasms are rare metastases to SCF. In this example of an epithelioid hemangioendothelioma, the malignant cells have large eccentrically placed nuclei with macronucleoli. Due to the rare nature of this lesion and a prominent epithelioid appearance, the diagnosis should be confirmed by immunostaining with vascular markers (Papanicolaou, high power).

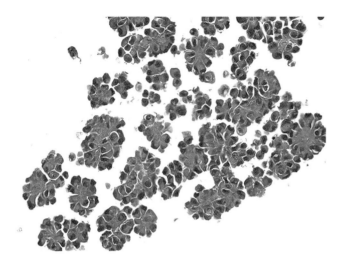

Fig. 5.51. *Epithelioid hemangioendothelioma. Pleural effusion.* Cell block section illustrates the characteristic "floweret" appearance of the neoplastic cells. Due to the reverse polarity, the nuclei are located at the outer edges of the cell cytoplasm creating this characteristic architecture (H & E, low power).

Sarcomas

- May mimic a variety of tumors
- Immunostaining is needed when pathognomonic features are absent

Sarcomatous Effusions – Some Facts

- *NEVER* present as occult metastases
- Objective of the cytologic examination is to:
  - Document the presence or absence of cancer
  - Confirm the morphologic resemblance to the known primary sarcoma
- *IMPERATIVE* to review/compare with the original resection specimen
- Perform ancillary studies

Sarcomas – Cytomorphologic Characteristics

- Large pleomorphic cells
- MFH, liposarcoma, undifferentiated embryonal sarcoma, MMMT
- Epithelioid/round cells
- Osteosarcoma, chondrosarcoma, clear cell sarcoma
- Small round blue cells
- Ewing's sarcoma/PNET, endometrial stromal sarcoma, embryonal rhabdomyosarcoma
- Spindle/fusiform cells
- Leiomyosarcoma, PNST

FIG. 5.52. *Epithelioid sarcoma. Pleural fluid.* In this rare example, the tumor cells show round to oval nuclei and prominent nucleoli, resembling an epithelial neoplasm. Diagnosis in such cases hinges upon the clinical history of a previous sarcoma as in most cases the phenotypic appearance can be nonspecific (Papanicolaou, high power).

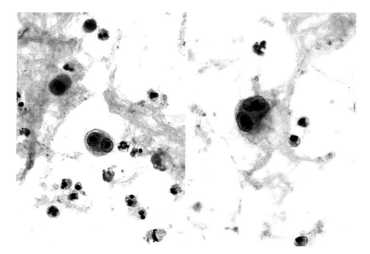

FIG. 5.53. *Clear cell sarcoma. Pericardial effusion.* This patient had a large ankle soft tissue mass resected a few months before this effusion was tapped. The malignant cells display binucleation with macronucleoli and a distinct paranuclear globoid inclusion (similar to a rhabdoid tumor) (Papanicolaou, high power).

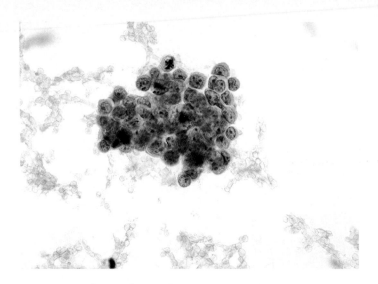

Fig. 5.54. *Endometrial stromal sarcoma, low grade. Peritoneal fluid.* A large fragment of high N/C ratio cells is seen. The cells barely display any cytoplasm and appear as mostly naked nuclei. A previous history of a uterine primary is extremely important. A CD10 immunostain would confirm the diagnosis (Papanicolaou, high power).

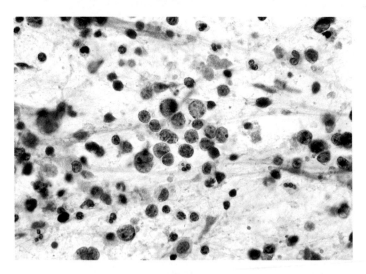

Fig. 5.55. *Endometrial stromal sarcoma, high grade. Peritoneal fluid.* In contrast to the previous example, this high-grade sarcoma shows numerous karyorrhectic nuclei and background necrosis (Papanicolaou, high power).

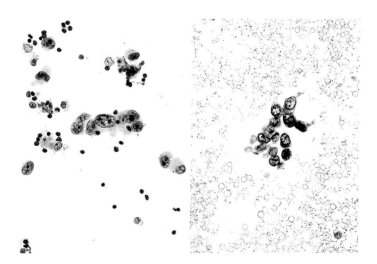

FIG. 5.56. *Leiomyosarcoma. Pleural effusion.* Very often, spindle cell sarcomas appear much more rounded (or "epithelioid") in SCF due to the prolonged
suspension of the malignant cells in a fluid environment. In this example of
leiomyosarcoma, the spindle cell morphology is lost despite the fact that primary leg sarcoma had fusiform nuclei. A confirmatory immunostain with
muscle-cell actin is shown on the right (Papanicolaou, high power).

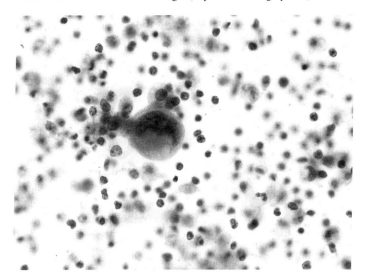

FIG. 5.57. *Malignant fibrous histiocytoma (MFH). Pleural fluid.* A pleomorphic multinucleated giant cell is visible in a background with extensive necrosis. A specific cytologic diagnosis is impossible in this case
without knowing the history of a known retroperitoneal MFH (Papanicolaou, high power).

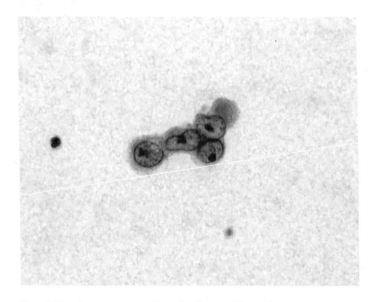

FIG. 5.58. *Osteosarcoma. Pleural effusion.* These high N/C ratio cells have vesicular nuclei and prominent nucleoli. The cytologic diagnosis would not have been possible without knowing the history of a lower femoral shaft osteosarcoma (Papanicolaou, high power).

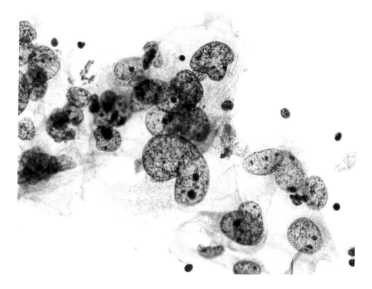

FIG. 5.59. *Undifferentiated embryonal sarcoma of liver. Peritoneal fluid.* This young child had a large liver tumor. The malignant cells seen here have extreme pleomorphism with large nuclei, macronucleoli, and fine wispy cytoplasm (Papanicolaou, high power).

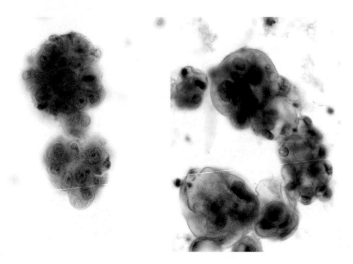

FIG. 5.60. Malignant mixed Mullerian tumor of uterus. *Ascitic fluid.* This pleomorphic tumor is attempting to form glandular structures. The cells display large nuclei, macronucleoli, and cytoplasmic vacuoles. Without the known history of a uterine MMMT, the cytomorphology would have been considered consistent with an adenocarcinoma. MMMT may also display sarcomatous components in SCF (Papanicolaou, high power).

Selected Reading

Abadi MA, Zakowski MF. Cytologic features of sarcomas in fluids. Cancer Cytopathol. 1998;84:71–6.

Blonk DI, Schaberg A, Willighagen RG. Enzyme cytochemistry of benign and malignant cells in pleural and peritoneal fluid. Acta Cytol. 1967;11(6):460–5.

Grefte JM, de Wilde PC, de Pol MR Salet-van, Tomassen M, Raaymakers-van Geloof WL, Bulten J. Improved identification of malignant cells in serous effusions using a small, robust panel of antibodies on paraffin-embedded cell suspensions. Acta Cytol. 2008;52(1):35–44.

Grunze H. The comparative diagnostic accuracy, efficiency and specificity of cytologic technics used in the diagnosis of malignant neoplasm in serous effusions of the pleural and pericardial cavities. Acta Cytol. 1964;8:150–63.

Hsu C. Cytologic detection of malignancy in pleural effusion: a review of 5,255 samples from 3,811 patients. Diagn Cytopathol. 1987;3(1):8–12.

Kim JH, Kim GE, Choi YD, Lee JS, Lee JH, Nam JH, Choi C. Immuno-cytochemical panel for distinguishing between adenocarcinomas and reactive mesothelial cells in effusion cell blocks. Diagn Cytopathol. 2009;37(4):258–61.

Longatto Filho A, Alves VA, Kanamura CT, Nonogaki S, Bortolan J, Lombardo V, Bisi H. Identification of the primary site of metastatic adenocarcinoma in serous effusions. Value of an immunocytochemical panel added to the clinical arsenal. Acta Cytol. 2002;46(4):651–8.

Longatto-Filho A, Bisi H, Bortolan J, Granja NV, Lombardo V. Cyto-logic diagnosis of metastatic sarcoma in effusions. Acta Cytol. 2003;47(2):317–8.

Pomjanski N, Grote HJ, Doganay P, Schmiemann V, Buckstegge B, Böck-ing A. Immunocytochemical identification of carcinomas of unknown primary in serous effusions. Diagn Cytopathol. 2005;33(5):309–15.

Sears D, Hajdu SI. The cytologic diagnosis of malignant neoplasms in pleural and peritoneal effusions. Acta Cytol. 1987;31(2):85–97.

Spieler P, Gloor F. Identification of types and primary sites of malignant tumors by examination of exfoliated tumor cells in serous fluids. Com-parison with the diagnostic accuracy on small histologic biopsies. Acta Cytol. 1985;29(5):753–67.

Westfall DE, Fan X, Marchevsky AM. Evidence-based guidelines to opti-mize the selection of antibody panels in cytopathology: pleural effusions with malignant epithelioid cells. Diagn Cytopathol. 2010;38(1):9–14.

6
Effusions in Children

Serous cavity effusions in children are usually related to infectious diseases, and malignant effusions are distinctly uncommon.
The latter, when seen, typically include malignant tumors of the
small round blue cell family such as neuroblastoma, nephroblastoma, Wilms' tumor, hepatoblastoma, and rhabdomyosarcoma. In
one large series (Wong et al. 1997), the incidence was lymphoma
and leukemia (52%), neuroblastoma (14%), Wilms' tumor (9%),
gonadal and extragonadal germ cell neoplasms (8%), bone and
soft tissue sarcomas (7%), epithelial neoplasms (5%), Ewing's
sarcoma/PNET (2%), and other neoplasms (3%). Cancers were
encountered in 47% of pleural fluids, 23% of ascitic fluids, 27% of
peritoneal washings, and 43% of pericardial fluids. Pleural fluids
were the most common specimen type and showed the highest pro-
portion of positivity. Others (Hallman and Geisinger) have shown
that the major diagnostic difficulty in interpreting pediatric effusion cytology is in distinguishing neoplasms of the small-cell type
from mononuclear inflammatory cells. The usefulness of peritoneal washings in pediatric patients is similar to that in adults.

S.Z. Ali and E.S. Cibas, *Serous Cavity Fluid and Cerebrospinal
Fluid Cytopathology*, Essentials in Cytopathology 10,
DOI 10.1007/ 978-1-4614-1776-7_6,
© Springer Science+Business Media, LLC 2012

Malignant Effusions in Children

- Small round blue cell tumors
  - Ewing's sarcoma/PNET
  - Wilms' tumor
  - Neuroblastoma
  - Embryonal rhabdomyosarcoma
  - DSRCT
  - Hepatoblastoma
- Hematologic neoplasms
  - Lymphomas and leukemias
- Other tumors
  - Extrarenal rhabdoid tumor

Malignant Effusions in Children – Cytomorphologic Findings (Figs. 6.1, 6.2, 6.3, 6.4, 6.5, 6.6, 6.7, 6.8, 6.9, 6.10, 6.11, 6.12, 6.13, 6.14 and 6.15)

- Small round blue cell tumors
  - Hypercellular, mostly single cells
  - Monotonous, small round blue cells
  - Rosetting and/or nuclear molding
  - Occasional mitoses, rare necrosis
- Hematologic neoplasms
  - See Chap. 8
- Extrarenal rhabdoid tumor
  - Large epithelioid cells
  - Eccentric nuclei with macronucleoli
  - Globular fibrillary cytoplasmic inclusions

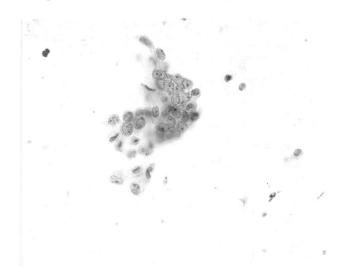

FIG. 6.1. *Neuroblastoma. Pleural fluid.* This case, prepared on a filter, essentially illustrates a population of primitive small round blue cells. The cytomorphology would generate a specific list of differential diagnosis in this age group. Additional immunostains are almost always needed. Neuroblastoma is a childhood tumor originating from sympathetic nervous system cells and represents one of the most common malignancies in early childhood. Neuroblastoma is a cancer with a heterogeneous profile and a prognosis ranging from near uniform survival to high risk for fatal demise. The expression of the MYCN oncogene is considered critical for progression of neuroblastoma (Papanicolaou, high power).

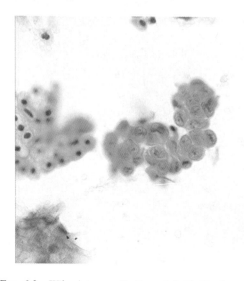

FIG. 6.2. *Wilms' tumor. Peritoneal fluid.* Similar to the previous case, fragments of small round *blue cells* are seen. Occasional cases of Wilms' tumor may also display better differentiated areas with tubular formations. Others have reported epithelial cells with three-dimensional aggregates with many cystic and tubular structures. Wilms' tumor, also known as nephroblastoma or renal embryoma, is the fifth most common pediatric malignancy, arising from the embryonal tissue of kidneys. This childhood cancer has an overall cure rate of over 85% (Papanicolaou, high power).

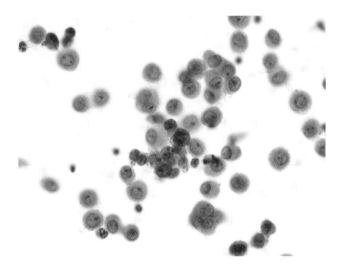

FIG. 6.3. *Ewing's sarcoma/PNET. Pleural fluid.* A distinct population of small round *blue cells* is seen in the *middle* of the field in the background of reactive mesothelial cells and histiocytes. Immunostaining with CD99 and bcl-2 would confirm the diagnosis in this case. SCFs are considered excellent samples for molecular and cytogenetic analysis in the small round blue cell tumors of the childhood, and such studies are occasionally required in difficult cases even after immunostaining has been performed. Ewing's sarcoma/PNET represents the second commonest primary osseous malignancy in adolescents and young adults (Papanicolaou, high power).

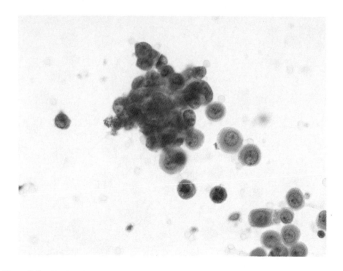

FIG. 6.4. *Ewing's sarcoma/PNET. Pleural fluid.* This tumor, due to tight nuclear molding, resembles a neuroendocrine carcinoma. However, due to the young age of the patient and additional immunostains, these cells were deemed consistent with Ewing's sarcoma/PNET. The tumor can occur in any bone in the body; the most common sites are the pelvis, thigh, lower leg, upper arm, and rib and can be extraskeletal (primarily arising in the soft tissues). The metastatic Ewing's sarcoma/PNET has an extremely poor prognosis. Despite aggressive treatment, 20–40% of patients with localized disease and almost 80% of patients with metastatic disease at presentation die of their disease (Papanicolaou, high power).

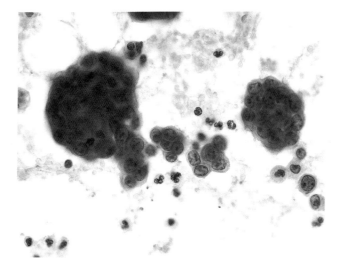

Fig. 6.5. *Renal medullary carcinoma. Pleural effusion.* This young patient had enlarged neck lymph nodes consistent with a metastatic disease. Additionally, the patient was sickle cell trait positive. Cytomorphology in this effusion strongly suggested an adenocarcinoma. However, due to the young age of the patient and the clinical history, this was reported as consistent with renal medullary carcinoma. Note the three-dimensional tumor cell fragments comprised of high N/C ratio malignant cells, nuclear hyperchromasia, and frequent mitoses (Papanicolaou, high power).

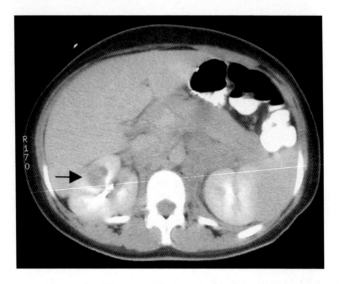

FIG. 6.6. *Renal medullary carcinoma. Radiologic imaging.* A transaxial CT scan at the level of the kidneys shows a large cystic right renal mass in this patient (arrow). Renal medullary carcinoma is a rare tumor that arises centrally in the renal medulla. Due to its rapid growth and invasion of the renal sinuses, it behaves very aggressively with nearly all patients dying of the disease within days to several months after the initial diagnosis. The mean duration of life after surgery is about 15 weeks. The *right* kidney is involved much more often than *left*.

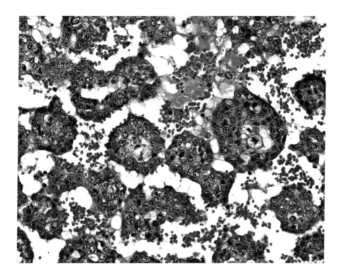

FIG. 6.7. *Renal medullary carcinoma. Pericardial effusion.* Cell block section in the previous case shows an aggressive phenotype with brisk mitoses and karyorrhexis. Luminal spaces suggest gland-like differentiation in this high-grade tumor. Cytologically, tumor cells display dark eosinophilic cytoplasm and nuclei with conspicuous and usually prominent nucleoli. The presence of rhabdoid-like cells has also been reported in some cases. Renal medullary carcinoma is typically seen in young patients with the sickle cell trait and rarely with sickle cell disease. The infiltrative pattern of growth of renal medullary carcinoma is in sharp contrast with renal cell carcinoma and Wilms' tumor, which grow by expansion (H & E, low power).

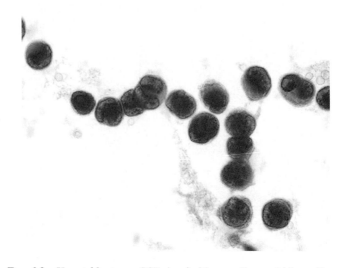

FIG. 6.8. *Hepatoblastoma. SCF.* A primitive small *round blue cell* neo-plasm is seen. However, with the history of a large hepatic mass in this young baby and an extremely high serum alpha fetoprotein, this case was adequately interpreted as metastatic hepatoblastoma. Without clinical history and serological information, a definitive diagnosis would not have been possible in this case as the morphological features are not specific for hepatoblastoma and any childhood small-cell tumor could show similar cellular characteristics. These limitations should always be kept in mind when interpreting the rare childhood malignancies. Although rare, hepatoblastoma accounts for two-thirds of malignant liver tumors in children. Patients with familial adenomatous polyposis (*FAP*) frequently develop hepatoblastomas. Complete surgical resection of the tumor at diagnosis, followed by adjuvant chemotherapy, is associated with 100% survival rates (Papanicolaou, high power).

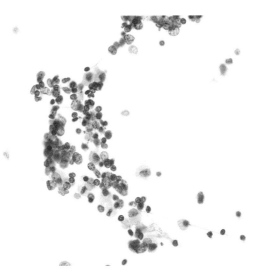

FIG. 6.9. *Intra-abdominal desmoplastic small-round-cell tumor (DSRCT). Peritoneal fluid.* Depicted is a dispersed population of small *round blue cells* with fine powdery chromatin and uniform round to oval nuclei. Intra-abdominal location and the young age favored this diagnosis, which was further confirmed in cell block sections with neuroendocrine markers and desmin. These patients may present with innumerable tumor nodules studding the entire peritoneal cavity. DSRCT is considered a multifocal disease. Metastases can be found in lung and liver. DSRCT is an aggressive intra-abdominal malignancy with excellent chemoresponsiveness, but relapse is frequent (Papanicolaou, low power).

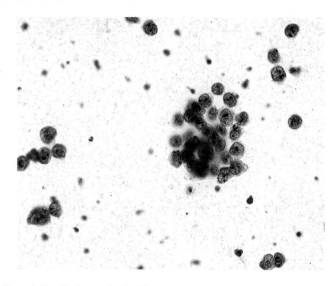

FIG. 6.10. *Embryonal rhabdomyosarcoma (RMS). Pleural effusion.* Loosely aggregated population of primitive small *round blue cells* is seen. In conjunction with the patient's previous history of a known RMS and immunostaining in the cell block sections with desmin and myogenin, this case was diagnosed as consistent with the above diagnosis. Rhabdomyosarcoma is the most frequent soft tissue sarcoma in children (Papanicolaou, high power).

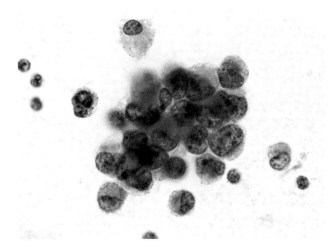

FIG. 6.11. *Embryonal rhabdomyosarcoma. Pleural effusion.* This filter preparation shows high N/C ratio cells with hyperchromatic nuclei. A diagnosis of RMS in the effusion is not possible without clinical history of the known primary and/or ancillary studies. The most common primary site of origin is head and neck with embryonal RMS being the most common histologic subtype. The 5-year survival rate is around 48% and depends on the primary site, histologic subtype, and size of the tumor at the time of presentation. The final clinical outcome for infants with RMS is less satisfactory than older children, and those aged 1–9 years have the best 5-year survival (Papanicolaou, high power).

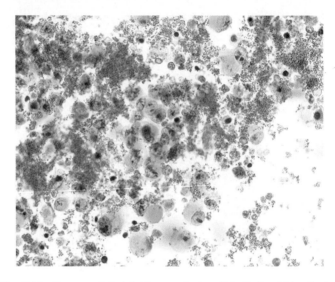

FIG. 6.12. *Extrarenal rhabdoid tumor. Pericardial effusion.* This effusion was tapped from a 2-week-old baby with a large chest wall mass. Presence of degenerated blood is a worrisome finding. The epithelioid malignant cells are singly dispersed with large nuclei and macronucleoli. Extrarenal rhabdoid tumor is a rare, highly aggressive tumor of childhood with a poor prognosis. It represents <1% of pediatric soft tissue malignancies, typically involving infants (Papanicolaou, low power).

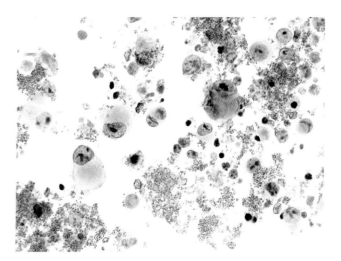

Fig. 6.13. *Extrarenal rhabdoid tumor. Pericardial effusion.* The classic "rhabdoid" morphology is evident here with large epithelioid cells with eccentric nuclei, single macronucleolus, and a whorled/globoid paranuclear cytoplasmic inclusion. Rhabdoid tumor frequently involves extrarenal sites such as the neck, abdomen, and paraspinal regions (Papanicolaou, high power).

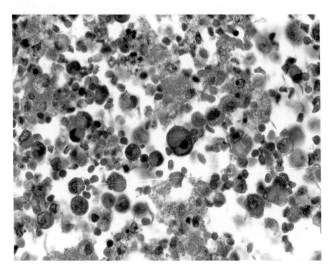

FIG. 6.14. *Extrarenal rhabdoid tumor. Pericardial effusion.* Cell block section illustrates the prominent rhabdoid appearance of the neoplastic cells. Note the characteristic macronucleoli. In an adult patient, differential diagnosis would also have included metastatic adenocarcinoma and mesothelioma. The effusion specimen in this case was also used to culture cells for karyotypic analysis and demonstrated the characteristic t(1;22) translocation (H & E, high power).

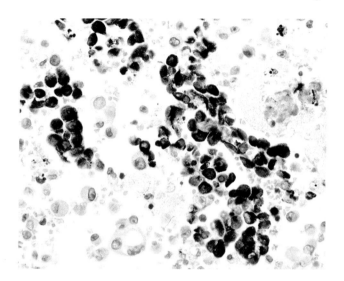

Fɪɢ. 6.15. *Extrarenal rhabdoid tumor. Pericardial effusion.* Cell block section shows strong immunostaining with EMA. Additionally, the tumor cells stained with desmin. Extrarenal RT is more common than either renal or CNS RTs, the latter observed in older patients. Concomitant CNS RTs are found in almost one-third of patients with extrarenal RT. Metastatic disease at diagnosis is present in more than half of the patients (high power).

Selected Reading

Crapanzano JP, Cardillo M, Lin O, Zakowski MF. Cytology of desmoplastic small round cell tumor. Cancer. 2002;96(1):21–31.

Dehner LP. A contemporary view of neoplasms in children. The pathologist's perspective. Pediatr Clin North Am. 1989;36(1):113–37.

Farr GH, Hajdu SI. Exfoliative cytology of metastatic neuroblastoma. Acta Cytol. 1972;16(3):203–6.

Geisinger KR, Hajdu SI, Helson L. Exfoliative cytology of nonlymphoreticular neoplasms in children. Acta Cytol. 1984;28(1):16–28.

Haddad MG, Silverman JF, Joshi VV, Geisinger KR. Effusion cytology in Burkitt's lymphoma. Diagn Cytopathol. 1995;12(1):3–7.

Hallman JR, Geisinger KR. Cytology of fluids from pleural, peritoneal and pericardial cavities in children. A comprehensive survey. Acta Cytol. 1994;38(2):209–17.

Helson L, Krochmal P, Hajdu SI. Diagnostic value of cytologic specimens obtained from children with cancer. Ann Clin Lab Sci. 1975;5(4): 294–7.

Perlman EJ, Ali SZ, Robinson R, Lindato R, Griffin CA. Infantile extrarenal rhabdoid tumor. Pediatr Dev Pathol. 1998;1(2):149–52.

Utine GE, Ozçelik U, Kiper N, Doğru D, Yalçn E, Cobanoğlu N, Pekcan S, Kara A, Cengiz AB, Ceyhan M, Seçmeer G, Göçmen A. Pediatric pleural effusions: etiological evaluation in 492 patients over 29 years. Turk J Pediatr. 2009;51(3):214–9.

Weir EG, Ali SZ. Hepatoblastoma: cytomorphologic characteristics in serious cavity fluids. Cancer. 2002;96(5):267–74.

Wong JW, Pitlik D, Abdul-Karim FW. Cytology of pleural, peritoneal and pericardial fluids in children. A 40-year summary. Acta Cytol. 1997;41(2):467–73.

7
Abdominopelvic Washings

Morphologic evaluation and appropriate characterization of neoplastic cells in peritoneal and pelvic fluids are important in the staging of patients with ovarian neoplasms. Peritoneal and/or pelvic washing specimens are submitted routinely for cytologic evaluation as part of the staging protocol for gynecologic tract and other abdominal cancers. Both benign conditions as well as malignant cells from a locally invasive tumor or a distant primary site can be observed in abdominopelvic washings (APW). Accurate pathologic evaluation and staging of the extent of the disease is important to determine the necessity for further therapy. One study highlighted the diagnostic problems encountered on cytologic evaluation as differentiating reactive mesothelial cells from low-grade malignancies, distinguishing between benign ovarian tumors, ovarian tumors of borderline malignancy, and low-grade ovarian malignancies; and potential false-positive diagnoses in endometriosis and endosalpingiosis. Another study included mesothelial cell hyperplasia, collagen balls, endometriosis, and endosalpingiosis as the most serious diagnostic pitfalls on peritoneal washing cytology in women who present with gynecologic lesions.

In a typical APW for a suspected gynecologic tract disease, approximately 200 cm^3 of sterile normal saline is instilled and

S.Z. Ali and E.S. Cibas, *Serous Cavity Fluid and Cerebrospinal Fluid Cytopathology*, Essentials in Cytopathology 10, DOI 10.1007/ 978-1-4614-1776-7_7,
© Springer Science+Business Media, LLC 2012

allowed to wash the uterus, tubes, ovaries, and cul-de-sac. The fluid is then aspirated, mixed with 1,000 units of heparin, and sent to the cytology laboratory. If the fluid is grossly bloody, lysing with a hemolytic agent (such as glacial acetic acid) often helps.

Benign Diseases (Figs. 7.1, 7.2, 7.3, 7.4, 7.5, 7.6, 7.7, 7.8, 7.9, 7.10, 7.11 and 7.12)

Endometriosis, endosalpingiosis, mesothelial proliferation, and hyperplasia (such as in cases of ovarian cystadenofibromas) are commonly diagnosed in APWs. The hallmarks of a washing specimen (as

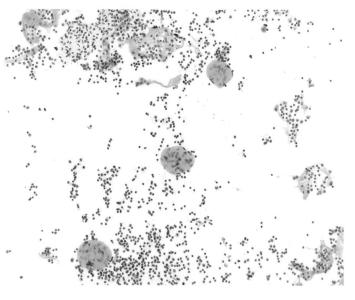

FIG. 7.1. *Collagen ball. Abdominopelvic washing.* Often considered a misnomer, these peculiar structures are a hallmark of abdominopelvic washing on cytology and are almost never seen in spontaneous effusions. Collagen balls have no clinical significance and likely represent the loose submesothelial matrix tissue which gets "rolled-up" with the adhered mesothelial cells due to physical trauma of the wash. Collagen balls tend to occur more commonly in pelvic than the rest of the abdominal washings and seem to arise from the surface of the ovaries (Papanicolaou, low power).

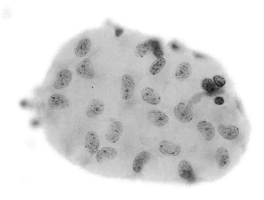

FIG. 7.2. *Collagen ball. Abdominopelvic washing.* This shows the *pale green* submesothelial matrix tissue with several benign mesothelial cell nuclei surrounding the core. These structures should not be confused with acini formations of a metastatic adenocarcinoma. Some have reported an unexplained sevenfold increase in the percentage of peritoneal washing samples with collagen balls, perhaps related to a better appreciation of this clinically unremarkable structure in routine cytology practice (Papanicolaou, high power).

opposed to spontaneous effusion or ascites) are the presence of large intact tissue fragments of benign mesothelium and/or the round to oval structures called "collagen balls." The presence of these two cellular components is explained by the physical lifting up of the fragile mesothelium from the underlying stroma to which these cells are only loosely adherent. The mesothelial fragments more commonly assume small- to large-sized monolayered fragments or linear fragments often referred to as "string of pearls." Collagen balls (a misnomer) are round to oval structures of varying sizes that appear pale green. The center (which appears amorphous) is surrounded by an attenuated lining of flattened mesothelium. The amorphous center does not contain collagen but is thought to consist of loose submesothelial matrix tissue which rolls up into balls due to the washing. Endometriosis in particular should always be included in the differential diagnosis of peritoneal effusions, or APWs, from women.

Endometriosis

- Young to middle-aged women, history of pelvic pain, can be asymptomatic, often ascites is presenting complaint
- Ovary is the most common site
- Often nonspecific cytologic findings of:
  - Bland-appearing endometrial cells, often in small tissue fragments, can be seen singly, but mostly small tight balls of epithelial cells, less often cells in syncytia and honeycombs
  - Psammoma bodies
  - Hemosiderin-laden macrophages are common and can predominate
  - Spindled stromal cells are rarely identified
  - Acute inflammatory cells (depending on the influence of hormonal levels)
- The appearance of the glandular component can be altered by hormonal and metaplastic changes, as well as cytologic atypia and hyperplasia
- CD10 immunostaining in cell block sections may help in the diagnosis by identifying stromal cells but is not routinely indicated

FIG. 7.4. *Endometriosis. Abdominopelvic washing.* This example beautifully illustrates a classic tight ball of endometrial glandular cells admixed with hemosiderin-laden macrophages. Few reactive mesothelial cells are also seen, which are a common accompaniment of endometriosis (Papanicolaou, high power).

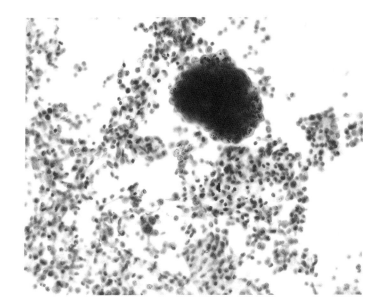

FIG. 7.3. *Endometriosis. Abdominopelvic washing.* A tight *ball-shaped* fragment of benign endometrial glandular epithelium is seen here. Note the small cell size, uniform nuclei lacking prominent nucleoli. No stromal cells or hemosiderin-laden macrophages are evident in this case. These two other cell types are not always needed in an effusion specimen to make the diagnosis of endometriosis as long as the clinical picture is consistent with the diagnosis (Papanicolaou, low power).

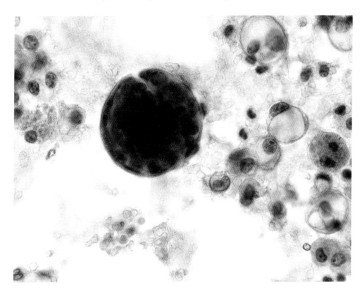

Endosalpingiosis

- Arises from secondary Mullerian system (pelvic and lower abdominal mesothelium)
- Young to middle-aged women
- Often asymptomatic
- Often large, epithelial fragments with tubal-type epithelium, indistinct ciliated border, smooth contours, often papillary-like, oval to elongated and stratified nuclei at the periphery
- Psammoma bodies
- No hemosiderin-laden macrophages

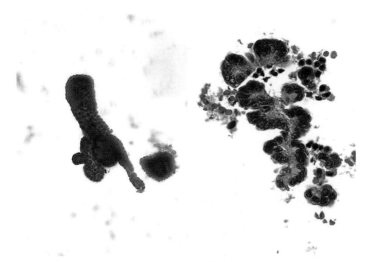

Fig. 7.5. *Endometriosis. Abdominopelvic washing.* A papillary-like fragment of endometrial glands containing a psammoma body in the middle (*left*). The corresponding cell block section nicely illustrates the benign endometrial tissue (*right*) (Papanicolaou and H & E, low power).

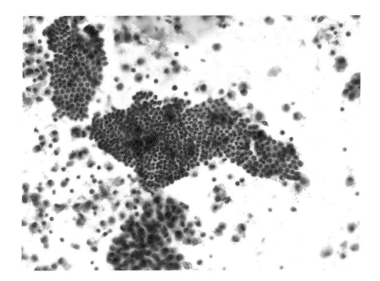

FIG. 7.6. *Endosalpingiosis. Abdominopelvic washing.* A large monolayered fragment of tubal-type epithelium with flat cuboidal cells forming a honeycombed architecture is depicted (Papanicolaou, low power).

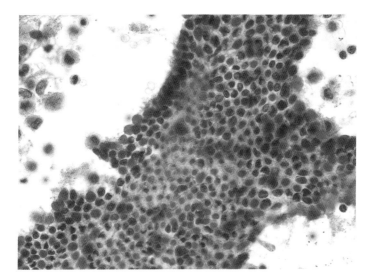

FIG. 7.7. *Endosalpingiosis. Abdominopelvic washing.* Higher magnification from the previous case shows focal ciliated border. Nuclei are enlarged and crowded with micronucleoli. Absence of significant atypia and lack of three dimensionality excluded a neoplastic process (Papanicolaou, high power).

158 7. Abdominopelvic Washings

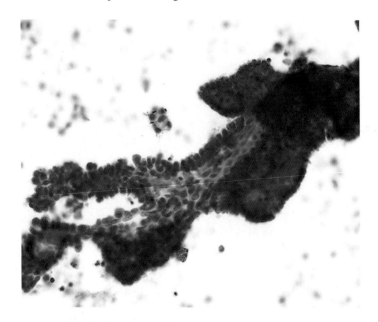

Fɪɢ. 7.8. *Endosalpingiosis. Abdominopelvic washing.* In this case, a large branching glandular fragment is seen with peripheral palisading of the nuclei which display short columnar- to cuboidal-type configuration. A psammoma body is also noticed at the *upper right* hand corner (Papanicolaou, low power).

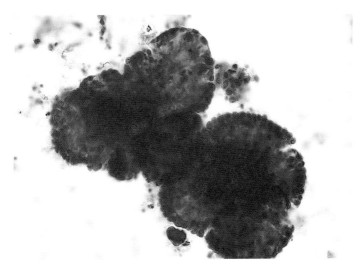

FIG. 7.9. *Endosalpingiosis. Abdominopelvic washing.* These round glandular fragments are lined by short columnar cells with focally ciliated borders, containing numerous psammoma bodies (Papanicolaou, high power).

FIG. 7.10. *Benign mesothelial proliferation with psammoma bodies.* Fragment of mesothelium with a crowded three-dimensional appearance. Note several partially intact psammoma bodies in the center of the fragment (Papanicolaou, high power).

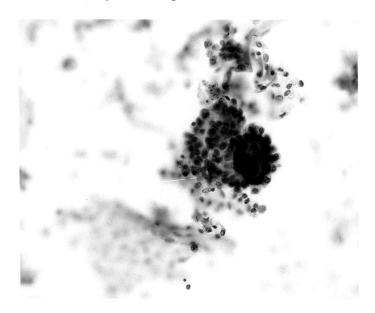

FIG. 7.11. *Benign mesothelial proliferation with psammoma bodies.* Seen here is benign-appearing mesothelium forming an acinus-like structure containing a large psammoma body. Mesothelial proliferation accompanies a number of nonneoplastic and neoplastic gynecologic tract conditions such as endometriosis, endosalpingiosis, and ovarian neoplasms (such as adenofibroma) (Papanicolaou, high power).

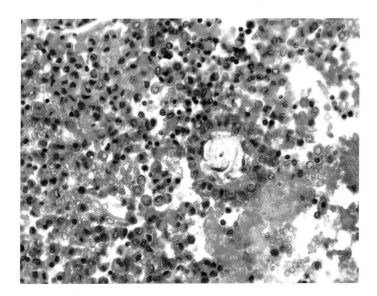

FIG. 7.12. *Benign mesothelial proliferation with psammoma bodies.* Cell block section illustrates an acinus-like structure occupied by a large partially intact psammoma body. This patient had a large ovarian adenofibroma, and the overlying mesothelium showed exuberant reactive hyperplasia (Papanicolaou, high power).

Malignant Diseases (Figs. 7.13, 7.14, 7.15, 7.16, 7.17, 7.18, 7.19, 7.20, 7.21, 7.22, 7.23, 7.24, 7.25, 7.26 and 7.27)

The cancers most often encountered in APWs are low-grade/borderline ovarian neoplasms (micropapillary serous), high-grade/serous ovarian carcinoma, and endometrial carcinomas.

Serous Borderline Tumors of the Ovary

- Young age, often the patient is pregnant
- Presence of a two-cell population
- Psammoma bodies
- Cytoplasmic vacuolization
- Smooth fragment contours
- High N/C ratios and coarse nuclear chromatin

Micropapillary Serous Carcinoma of the Ovary

- A proliferative serous ovarian neoplasm that often lacks destructive infiltrative growth but behaves like a low-grade invasive carcinoma
- Displays a characteristic histologic architecture consisting of a filigree pattern of highly complex micropapillae arising directly from large, bulbous papillary structures
- Can be associated with invasive peritoneal implants and, in these cases, the disease is likely to be progressive and fatal
- Cytomorphologic features
  - Small but well-formed papillary fragments (generally <30 cells)
  - Monotonous, relatively small, orderly arranged epithelial cells, with hyperchromatic nuclei often with multiple nucleoli
  - Occasionally, larger papillary fragments, which have a well-formed fibrovascular core
  - Prominent peripheral palisading of the nuclei with focal hob nailing of the nuclear contours, giving the fragments an undulating outer edge
  - Single, large atypical cells seldom present and seen in less than one-half of cases
  - Psammoma bodies are commonly present

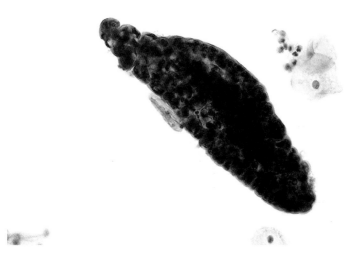

FIG. 7.13. *Micropapillary serous carcinoma of the ovary. Abdominopelvic washing.* A well-defined fragment of glandular epithelium is seen. Notice the fine papillary-like architecture, small cell size with nuclei lacking prominent nucleoli. In cases where a definitive cytologic diagnosis is not possible, it is better to wait an extra day and correlate the findings with the histology of the resected lesion (as most of the abdominopelvic washings are intraoperative procedures and are accompanied by a concurrent tissue resection) (Papanicolaou, low power).

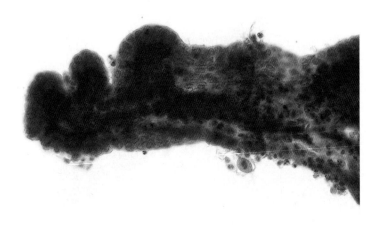

FIG. 7.14. *Micropapillary serous carcinoma of the ovary. Abdominopelvic washing.* A beautiful illustration of the fine finger-like papillary architecture of the tumor with the center containing what appears to be a fibrovascular core. Some peripheral palisading of the small cuboidal nuclei is visible at the top of the fragment (Papanicolaou, low power).

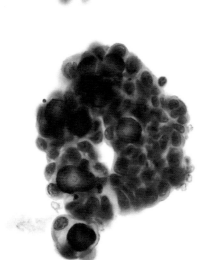

FIG. 7.15. *Micropapillary serous carcinoma of the ovary. Abdominopelvic washing.* Abundant mesothelial proliferation accompanies this tumor as evident here along with numerous small psammoma bodies (Papanicolaou, high power).

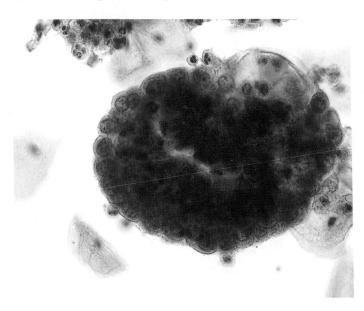

Fɪɢ. 7.16. *Micropapillary serous carcinoma of the ovary. Abdominopel-*
vic washing. Higher magnification shows the three-dimensional acinar-
like arrangement with uniform small cuboidal cells lacking nucleoli
(Papanicolaou, high power).

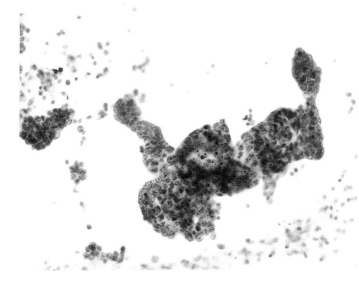

FIG. 7.17. *High-grade serous carcinoma of the ovary.* In contrast to micropapillary carcinoma, a high-grade serous carcinoma of the ovary shows a much higher cellularity with larger tissue fragments displaying a more complex architecture. Macronucleoli are hard to miss even at this low magnification (Papanicolaou, low power).

High-Grade Papillary Serous Carcinoma of the Ovary

- One of the most common epithelial tumor diagnoses of the ovary
- Primary mode of dissemination in ovarian carcinoma is intraperitoneal spread
- 5-year survival of 70% if confined to ovary; drops to 25% if it involves peritoneum
- Cytomorphologic features
  - Larger papillary fragments (generally >30 cells)
  - Disorderly placed pleomorphic, hyperchromatic cells, often with single prominent nucleoli
  - Papillary tissue fragments have a more complex, elaborate arborizing architecture
  - Pronounced nuclear crowding and pleomorphism with relatively larger round to oval-shaped nuclei. Nuclei show a distinct vesicular chromatin texture, often with single atypical-appearing nucleoli
  - Peripheral palisading of the nuclei rarely observed, in contrast to the MPSC specimens. Single large tumor cells exhibiting eccentrically placed atypical nuclei or multinucleation present in high concentration
- Immunostaining – WT-1 (78%), CA-125 (78%), CK 5/6 (55%), and D2-40 (23%)

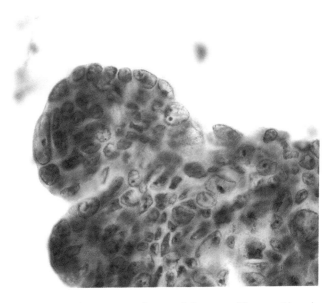

FIG. 7.18. *High-grade serous carcinoma of the ovary.* Pleomorphic epithelial cells with significant anisonucleosis, open chromatin, and macronucleoli are seen. High-grade serous carcinoma is fairly easy to diagnose on abdominopelvic washings as opposed to low-grade or borderline tumors (Papanicolaou, high power).

Psammomatous Effusions

Psammoma bodies (PBs) are encountered only rarely in SCFs. Psammomatous effusions are much more common in abdominal than pleural or pericardial cavities and in general observed more often in female patients undergoing intraoperative abdominopelvic washings. Although their presence in certain neoplasms of thyroid, ovary, lung, brain, etc., is established, their significance in SCF is not well understood. PBs are concentrically laminated calcific spherules that occasionally appear cracked on smears, surrounded by cells, and often appear either acidophilic or basophilic on Papanicolaou stain. PBs usually are associated with papillary neoplasms of various organs as well as a variety of benign conditions such as the use of intrauterine devices, oral contraceptives, endosalpingiosis, endometriosis, endometritis, and many others. The presence of PBs in fine

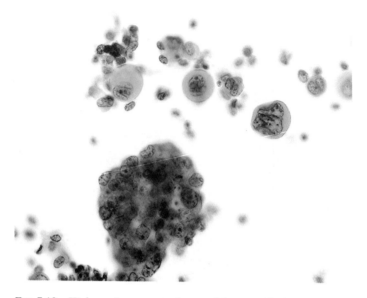

FIG. 7.19. *High-grade serous carcinoma of the ovary.* In this case, a large three-dimensional tissue fragment is evident with crowded and pleomorphic nuclei showing macronucleoli. Additionally, a few single malignant cells are present as well (Papanicolaou, low power).

needle aspiration of certain neoplasms, such as papillary thyroid carcinoma, ovarian papillary serous carcinoma, bronchioloalveolar carcinoma, meningioma, and others, is well established and is considered to be diagnostically significant. In one of the largest series (see the table below), the incidence was 3.7%. Of all PBs, 91% were seen in peritoneal fluid, 8.1% in pleural, and 0.81% in pericardial fluids. However, all cases of pleural and pericardial effusions with PBs were malignant (carcinomas of the thyroid, lung, and ovary) compared with 55.4% of peritoneal fluid (carcinoma of the ovary and uterus and mesothelioma). In 36.6% of peritoneal fluid with PB, the follow-up diagnoses were benign (ovarian cystadenoma/cystadenofibroma, papillary mesothelial hyperplasia, endosalpingiosis, endometriosis, and other miscellaneous benign diagnoses).

Cytomorphologically, PBs in SCFs are round, mostly intact structures with easily identifiable concentric laminations with a pale reddish coloration on Papanicolaou staining. They are almost always

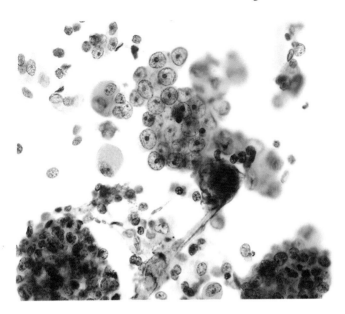

FIG. 7.20. *High-grade serous carcinoma of the ovary.* Depicted is a population of almost naked nuclei with open chromatin and macronucleoli. Occasionally, when the patient has more than one primary site, a positive immunostaining with WT-1 in the cell block sections is extremely helpful (Papanicolaou, high power).

observed in association with the cellular component. Only rarely are isolated PBs noted in the slide background. In benign lesions such as endosalpingiosis or endometriosis, the PBs are well formed and easily discernible structures and are well contained within the glandular lumina. The lining epithelial cells are observed to be well polarized around the periphery of the fragments. In cases of cystadenofibroma of the ovaries and benign mesothelial hyperplasia, PBs are noted to be associated with small papillary-like fragments of mesothelium. In benign lesions, the number of PBs is noted to range from rare (one to two) to few (three to five). However, in cases of cancers, the number of PBs usually is higher (greater than five), such as in ovarian carcinoma. Paraffin-embedded cell block sections offer a better visualization of the PBs. However, in the majority of cases, the PBs are observed to be shattered structures that still were associated with the cells of concern.

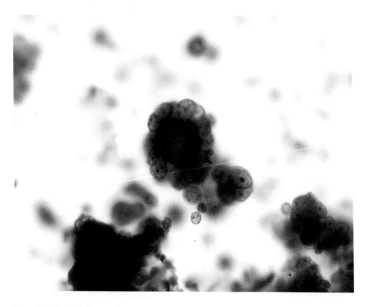

FIG. 7.21. *High-grade serous carcinoma of the ovary.* Malignant cells accompanied by a well-formed psammoma body. High-grade papillary serous carcinoma of the ovary is known to harbor abundant psammoma bodies (Papanicolaou, high power).

Psammomatous Effusions

- General incidence in SCFs   3.7%
  - Abdominal (91%)   Percentage malignant – 63%
  - Pleural (8%)   Percentage malignant – 100%
  - Pericardial (0.8%)   Percentage malignant – 100%
- Malignant abdominal effusions with psammoma bodies
  - Carcinoma of ovary or endometrium and MMMT
- Thirty-seven percent of abdominal effusions with psammoma bodies are benign
  - Endosalpingiosis, endometriosis, papillary mesothelial hyperplasia, cystadenoma/adenofibroma

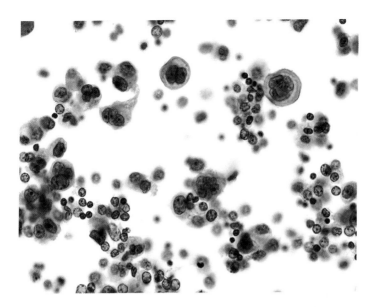

FIG. 7.22. *High-grade serous carcinoma of the ovary.* Another case which was almost exclusively comprised of singly dispersed pleomorphic malignant cells with frequent multinucleation. Background contains reactive mesothelial cells and histiocytes (Papanicolaou, high power).

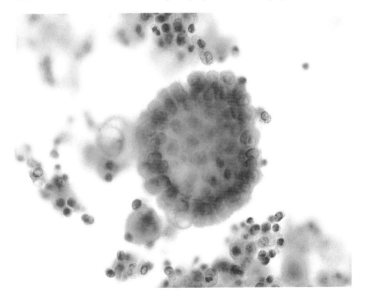

FIG. 7.23. *Serous surface papillary adenocarcinoma. Peritoneal washing.* A large truly three-dimensional tumor fragment seen here is comprised of high N/C ratio cuboidal cells. The center appears hollow and suggests a lumen formation (Papanicolaou, high power).

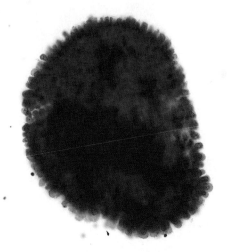

F<small>IG</small>. 7.24. *Serous surface papillary adenocarcinoma. Peritoneal washing.* In this case, the large tumor fragment shows prominent hob nailing of the outer edge due to enlarged nuclei. The center seems to contain psammoma bodies (Papanicolaou, low power).

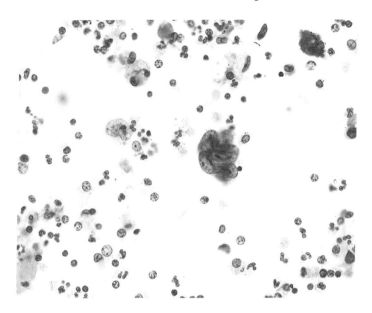

FIG. 7.25. *Serous borderline tumor of the ovary. Abdominopelvic washing.* The diagnosis of this tumor is often quite challenging. Although these pleomorphic tumor cells suggest a high-grade carcinoma, the follow-up diagnosis was a borderline serous tumor. Cytohistologic correlation is imperative to avoid misdiagnosis in such cases (Papanicolaou, high power).

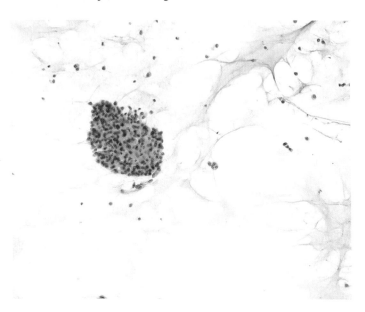

FIG. 7.26. *Pseudomyxoma peritonei, appendiceal primary. Peritoneal washing.* Abundant thin mucin containing a fragment of benign-appearing glandular epithelium is pictured. Presence of extensive mucin is a highly abnormal finding in an abdominal fluid even when the glandular component is missing and should raise a serious possibility of a low-grade mucinous neoplasm (Papanicolaou, low power).

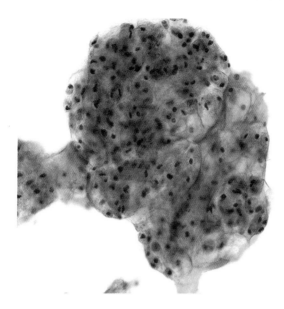

FIG. 7.27. *Pseudomyxoma peritonei, appendiceal primary. Peritoneal washing.* A large fragment of what appears to be muciphages trapped within a ball of thick mucin. No distinct glandular epithelium was identified in this case despite repeated tapping. The patient was found to have a small appendiceal mucin-producing neoplasm (Papanicolaou, high power).

Selected Reading

Cheng L, Wolf NG, Rose PG, Rodriguez M, Abdul-Karim FW. Peritoneal washing cytology of ovarian tumors of low malignant potential: correlation with surface ovarian involvement and peritoneal implants. Acta Cytol. 1998;42(5):1091–4.

Covell JL, Carry JB, Feldman PS. Peritoneal washings in ovarian tumors. Potential sources of error in cytologic diagnosis. Acta Cytol. 1985;29(3):310–6.

Mulvany N. Cytohistologic correlation in malignant peritoneal washings. Analysis of 75 malignant fluids. Acta Cytol. 1996;40(6):1231–9.

Ravinsky E. Cytology of peritoneal washings in gynecologic patients. Diagnostic criteria and pitfalls. Acta Cytol. 1986;30(1):8–16.

Sadeghi S, Ylagan LR. Pelvic washing cytology in serous borderline tumors of the ovary using ThinPrep: are there cytologic clues to detecting tumor cells? Diagn Cytopathol. 2004;30(5):313–9.

Selvaggi SM. Diagnostic pitfalls of peritoneal washing cytology and the role of cell blocks in their diagnosis. Diagn Cytopathol. 2003;28(6): 335–41.

Sneige N, Fanning CV. Peritoneal washing cytology in women: diagnostic pitfalls and clues for correct diagnosis. Diagn Cytopathol. 1992;8(6):632–40.

Stowell SB, Wiley CM, Perez-Reyes N, Powers CN. Cytologic diagnosis of peritoneal fluids. Applicability to the laparoscopic diagnosis of endometriosis. Acta Cytol. 1997;41(3):817–22.

Ziselman EM, Harkavy SE, Hogan M, West W, Atkinson B. Peritoneal washing cytology. Uses and diagnostic criteria in gynecologic neoplasms. Acta Cytol. 1984;28(2):105–10.

Zuna RE, Mitchell ML, Mulick KA, Weijchert WM. Cytohistologic correlation of peritoneal washing cytology in gynecologic disease. Acta Cytol. 1989;33(3):327–36.

8
Lymphocytic Effusions

Lymphocytes are commonly present in any SCF, admixed with mesothelial cells and histiocytes. When a predominant population of lymphocytes is observed, a careful evaluation of the morphologic features should permit distinction between a reactive process and lymphoproliferative disorder. However, in effusions where a large amount of small mature lymphocytes are encountered, a statement should be added to the cytologic report stating the diagnostic possibilities. Predominant lymphocytosis in an effusion caused by small mature lymphocytes can be seen in cases of an underlying tuberculosis (such as in the lung), a low-grade lymphoproliferative disorder, or an occult malignancy. In cases where a lymphoproliferative process is suspected, it is best to send a fresh portion of SCF for flow cytometric analysis. It is agreed that serous cavity involvement by a low-grade lymphoma is notoriously difficult to differentiate from a reactive process on cytopathology alone. Several studies have demonstrated the sensitivity of flow analysis when morphologic evaluation alone cannot provide a conclusive diagnosis of lymphoma.

S.Z. Ali and E.S. Cibas, *Serous Cavity Fluid and Cerebrospinal Fluid Cytopathology*, Essentials in Cytopathology 10, DOI 10.1007/ 978-1-4614-1776-7_8,
© Springer Science+Business Media, LLC 2012

Chronic Inflammatory Process vs. Lymphoma/Leukemia (Figs. 8.1, 8.2, 8.3, 8.4, 8.5, 8.6 and 8.7)

- Cytologic features
- Ancillary techniques
- Immunostaining
- Flow cytometry
- Cytogenetics and molecular studies

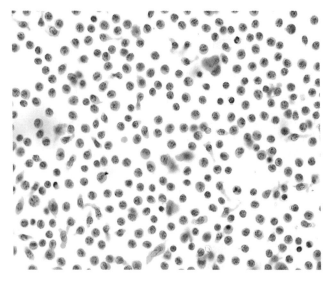

FIG. 8.1. *Tuberculous pleuritis.* This SCF shows a predominant population of small mature lymphocytes. No other abnormality was noted; however, the suspicion of TB or a lymphoproliferative disorder was raised on cytology. Follow-up serosal biopsy showed granulomatous inflammation (Papanicolaou, high power).

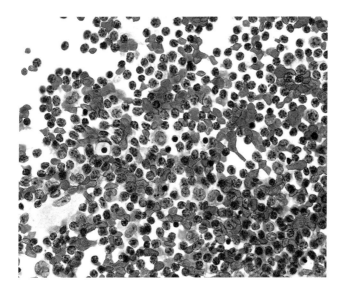

F<small>IG</small>. 8.2. *Tuberculous pleuritis.* Lymphocytosis comprised of small mature lymphocytes is seen. No granulomas or any other evidence of TB was noticed in this SCF. Immunostaining confirmed the T-cell lineage of these lymphocytes (Papanicolaou, high power).

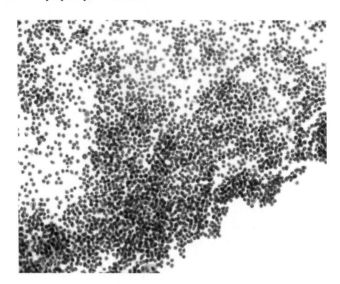

FIG. 8.3. *Reactive lymphocytosis. Ascitic fluid.* Pictured is hypercellularity due to an overabundance of small mature-appearing lymphocytes. Only rare mesothelial cells were present in this case (Papanicolaou, low power).

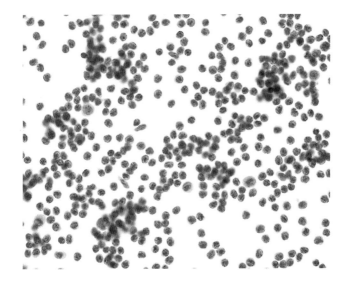

FIG. 8.4. *Reactive lymphocytosis. Ascitic fluid.* These cells have the characteristics of small mature lymphocytes; however, the possibility of involvement by a low-grade lymphomatous process (such as CML/SLL) is often difficult to exclude without immunostaining with B- and T-cell markers. Occasionally, a flow cytometric analysis is required if the clinical presentation is indicative of lymphoma/leukemia (Papanicolaou, high power).

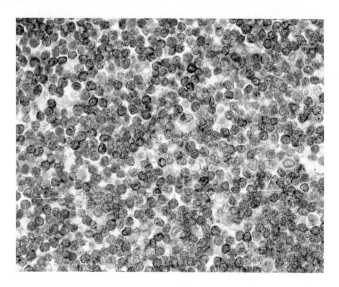

FIG. 8.5. *Reactive lymphocytosis. Ascitic fluid.* A diffuse immunolabeling in this cell block section from the above case with CD3 indicating a T-cell lineage consistent with a reactive process (high power).

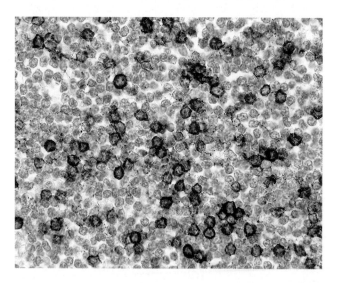

FIG. 8.6. *Reactive lymphocytosis. Ascitic fluid.* Cell block section displays only a few B cells as indicated by immunolabeling with CD20 (high power).

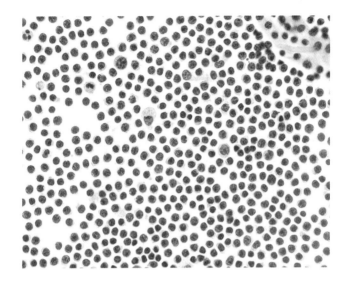

FIG. 8.7. *Reactive lymphocytosis. Ascitic fluid.* The uniform appearance of lymphocytes in this case prompted a flow cytometric analysis, which was consistent with a reactive polyclonal process despite the cytologic atypia present (nuclear monomorphism, nucleoli, etc.) (Papanicolaou, high power).

The role of flow cytometry (FC) in the diagnosis of lymphoid lesions by fine needle aspiration (FNA) is well established. However, studies evaluating the usefulness of FC in SCF are few. Malignant lymphomas may present as an effusion, but more often involve serous cavities secondarily. In a patient with malignant lymphoma, the accurate diagnosis of SCF constitutes part of the staging procedure and as such influences treatment decisions. The presence of a small population of malignant lymphoid cells may be difficult to detect on cytomorphology alone, especially if they are admixed with background reactive lymphoid cells as often seen in effusion samples. Cytomorphology combined with flow cytometry results in a substantial reduction of nondefinitive diagnoses in SCF specimens.

Role of Flow Cytometry as an Adjunct to Cytomorphologic Analysis

---

- 3 or 4 color analysis
- CD45, CD71, CD33, CD22, CD19, CD20, Kappa, Lambda, CD5, CD3, CD10, CD56
- 17% (16/96) – significant modification of pre-flow diagnosis[a]
- Cannot diagnose Hodgkin's lymphoma

---

[a]Czader and Ali, Diagn Cytopathol, 2003

Other studies have shown utility of molecular genetics in the diagnosis of lymphoid-rich effusions by using PCR and Southern blot analysis to assess B- and T-cell clonality (Mihaescu et al. 2002).

Malignant Effusions (Figs. 8.8, 8.9, 8.10, 8.11, 8.12, 8.13, 8.14, 8.15, 8.16, 8.17, 8.18, 8.19, 8.20, 8.21, 8.22, 8.23, 8.24, 8.25 and 8.26)

Serous cavity effusions are a common finding in malignant lymphomas. Pleural effusions are seen in 20–30% of all lymphomas (non-Hodgkin's and Hodgkin's) and uncommonly in peritoneal and pericardial cavities. Among the lymphoma subtypes, T-cell neoplasms, especially the lymphoblastic lymphomas, more frequently involve the serous fluids (Das). It is postulated that thoracic duct obstruction and impaired lymphatic drainage are the primary mechanisms for pathogenesis of pleural effusion in Hodgkin's lymphoma, and direct pleural infiltration is the predominant cause in NHL (Das). There is wide variation in the rate of positive cytologic findings of NHL in pleural effusion (22.2–94.1%).

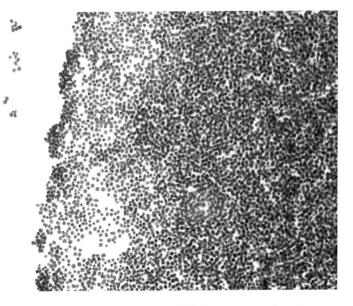

FIG. 8.8. *Large B-cell lymphoma in SCF.* A pure population of monomorphic lymphocytes is seen. No other cell type was appreciated in this peritoneal effusion (Papanicolaou, low power).

- Single cells
- Morphology varies according to the subtype
- Ancillary techniques (e.g., flow cytometry) are needed for definitive classification
- Differential diagnosis
  - Breast lobular carcinoma
  - Poorly differentiated carcinomas
  - Benign lymphocyte-rich effusions (e.g., TB)

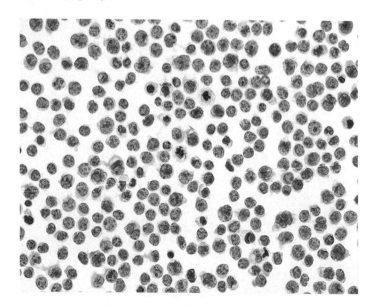

FIG. 8.9. *Large B-cell lymphoma in SCF.* Note the cellular monotony, irregular nuclear outlines, occasional prominent nucleoli, and numerous karyorrhectic bodies. Additionally, a flow cytometric analysis was consistent with an aggressive phenotype (Papanicolaou, high power).

Primary Effusion Lymphoma

- Rare form of non-Hodgkin's lymphoma seen frequently in HIV-positive patients
- Characterized by the development of effusion in one or more body cavities with no tumor masses and a positive human herpesvirus-8 (HHV-8) status
- Morphologically shares features of large-cell immunoblastic and anaplastic large-cell lymphoma
- Carries a very poor prognosis
- Malignant cells have a null phenotype but are believed to be of B-cell origin
- Detection of HHV-8 is an important confirmatory test

- High level of IL-6 in tumor cells, which aids in the diagnosis and could be a potential target for therapy
- Cytomorphologic features
  - High-grade lymphoma with round nuclei, prominent nucleoli, and abundant basophilic cytoplasm
  - Many cells have immunoblastic features; some display plasmocytoid differentiation
  - Numerous mitotic figures

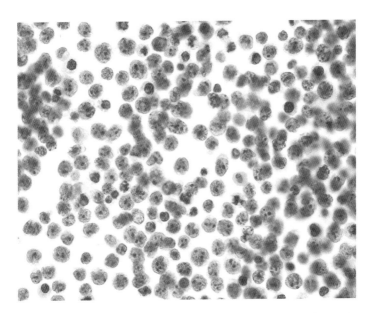

FIG. 8.10. *Large B-cell lymphoma in SCF.* This ascitic fluid is diagnostic of an aggressive large-cell lymphoma. In such cases where cytomorphology is diagnostic and the patient has a known history, further ancillary testing may not be needed. Note markedly irregular nuclear envelopes, prominent nucleoli, and extensive karyorrhexis (Papanicolaou, high power).

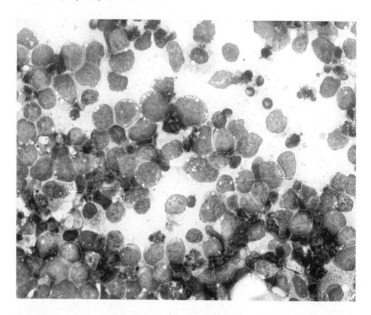

FIG. 8.11. *Burkitt's lymphoma.* This ascitic fluid shows malignant cells with finely granular chromatin, lack of nucleoli, and fine cytoplasmic vacuoles. Numerous mitoses are evident. Focal nuclear molding in an air-dried smear is usually an artifact and may lead to an erroneous diagnosis of a high-grade neuroendocrine carcinoma (Diff-Quik, high power).

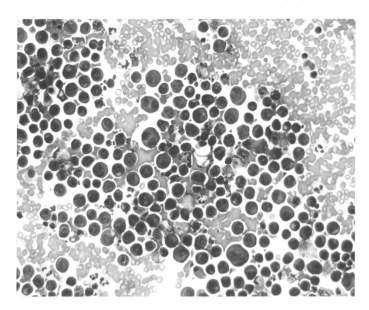

FIG. 8.12. *Primary effusion lymphoma.* Pleural fluid shows large populations of malignant lymphocytes with large nuclei, prominent nucleoli, frequent binucleation, and relatively abundant basophilic cytoplasm (Diff-Quik, high power).

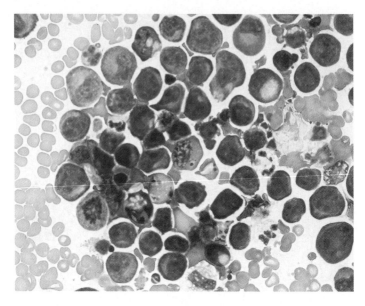

FIG. 8.13. *Primary effusion lymphoma.* Malignant characteristics are more obvious in this lymphoid population with nuclei having single or multiple nucleoli and mitoses. Abundance of cytoplasm is unusual in lymphoid malignancy and should raise the possibility of PEL in the right clinic-radiologic setting (Diff-Quik, high power).

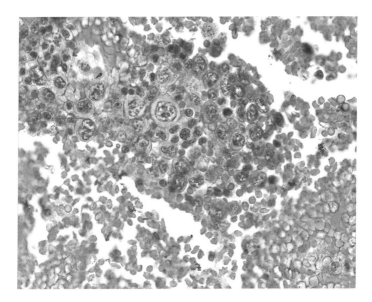

FIG. 8.14. *Primary effusion lymphoma.* Cell block section shows a high-grade malignancy. Cells are relatively large and show abundant cytoplasm and frequent binucleation. Pleomorphism and prominent nucleoli cause this tumor to resemble an anaplastic large-cell (Ki-1) lymphoma. Immunostains are usually extremely helpful in such cases (H & E, high power).

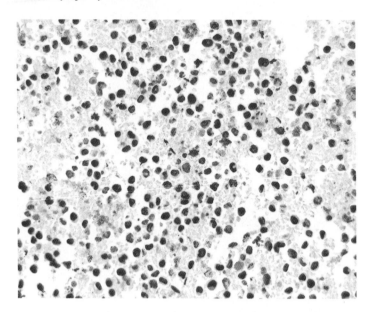

FIG. 8.15. *Primary effusion lymphoma.* Immunolabeling with HHV-8 in a cell block section shows diffuse and strong nuclear reaction (low power).

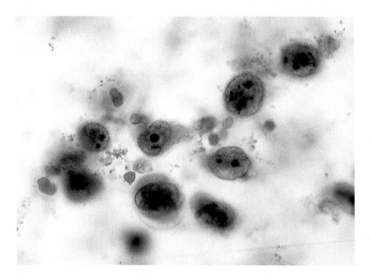

FIG. 8.16. *Anaplastic large-cell (Ki-1) lymphoma. Pleural effusion.* Pleomorphic malignant cells are difficult to interpret as lymphoid due to the large size, macronucleoli, and anisonucleosis (Papanicolaou, high power).

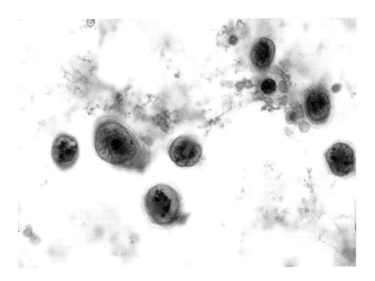

FIG. 8.17. *Anaplastic large-cell (Ki-1) lymphoma. Pleural effusion.* In addition to the extreme pleomorphism, cells in the photograph illustrate the so-called horseshoe-shaped or wreath-like nuclei characteristic of a Ki-1 lymphoma (Papanicolaou, high power).

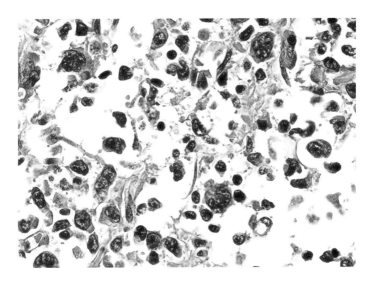

FIG. 8.18. *Anaplastic large-cell (Ki-1) lymphoma. Pleural effusion.* Cell block section displays extreme pleomorphism, markedly irregular nuclear contours, some spindled cells, and the characteristic "wreath-like" nuclei (H & E, high power).

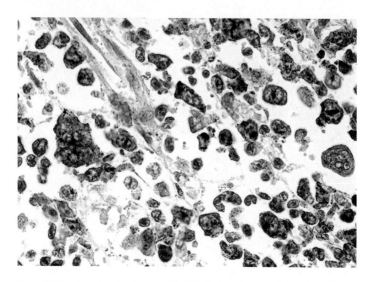

FIG. 8.19. *Anaplastic large-cell (Ki-1) lymphoma. Pleural effusion.* Immunoperoxidase staining is diffusely and strongly positive for CD30 (high power).

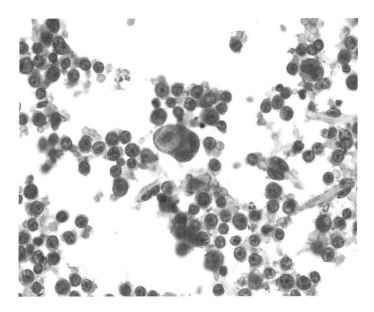

FIG. 8.20. *Plasma cell myeloma. Pleural effusion.* Neoplastic plasma cells with prominent nucleoli and frequent binucleation are pictured. A large pleomorphic cell is present in the middle of the field. Morphologic kinship with plasma cell differentiation is still retained as most nuclei are eccentrically placed in the cell cytoplasm and display speckled chromatin (Papanicolaou, high power).

FIG. 8.21. *Plasma cell myeloma. Pericardial effusion.* In these malignant cells, the only helpful clue is the eccentric nuclear placement. Without immunostaining or prior history, this would be a difficult case to diagnose as plasma cell myeloma (Papanicolaou, high power).

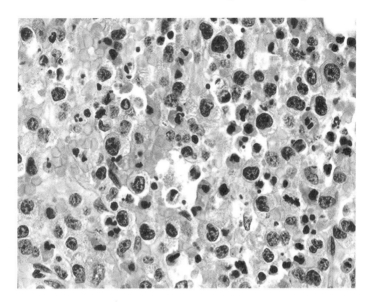

FIG. 8.22. *Plasma cell myeloma. Pericardial effusion.* Cell block section shows pleomorphic plasma cells with macronucleoli and abundant karyorrhexis. There is hardly any morphologic resemblance to plasma cells in this particular case (H & E, high power).

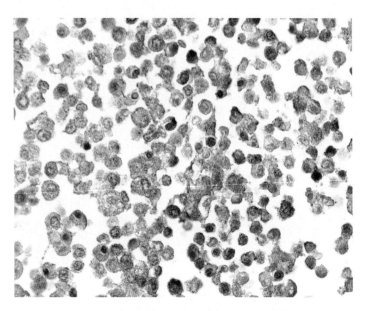

FIG. 8.23.   *Plasma cell myeloma. Pericardial effusion.* Cell block section shows strong and diffuse reactivity with CD138 consistent with plasma cell differentiation (high power).

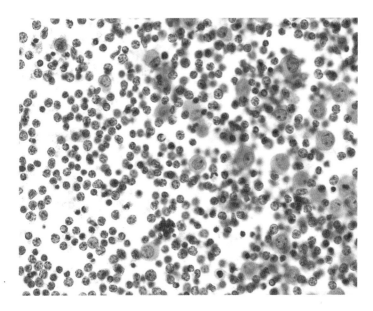

FIG. 8.24. *T-cell acute lymphoblastic leukemia. Pleural effusion.* Malignant small lymphocytes with blastoid morphology and few background reactive mesothelial cells are seen (Papanicolaou, high power).

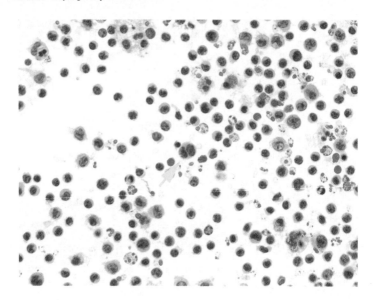

FIG. 8.25. *Hodgkin's lymphoma. Pleural fluid.* A classic Reed-Sternberg cell is observed (*arrow*) in a background of polymorphous lymphocytes and few eosinophils. A history of the disease is almost always known (Papanicolaou, high power).

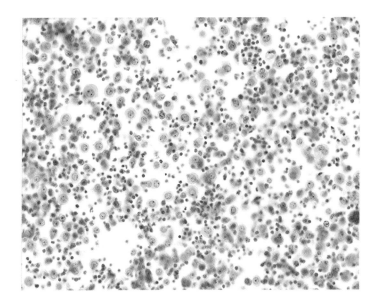

FIG. 8.26. *T-cell-rich B-cell lymphoma. Peritoneal fluid.* These cases are harder to diagnose on morphology due to a large population of mature T lymphocytes diluting the phenotypically abnormal and neoplastic B lymphocytes. This case was initially deemed reactive; however, flow analysis showed a small clonal population of malignant B cells (Papanicolaou, low power).

Selected Reading

Bangerter M, Hildebrand A, Griesshammer M. Combined cytomorphologic and immunophenotypic analysis in the diagnostic workup of lymphomatous effusions. Acta Cytol. 2001;45(3):307–12.

Chen LM, Hwang WS. Myeloma with pleural involvement. Acta Cytol. 1991;35(3):372–3.

Czader M, Ali SZ. Flow cytometry as an adjunct to cytomorphologic analysis of serous effusions. Diagn Cytopathol. 2003;29(2):74–8.

Das DK, Gupta SK, Ayyagari S, Bambery PK, Datta BN, Datta U. Pleural effusions in non-Hodgkin's lymphoma. A cytomorphologic, cytochemical and immunologic study. Acta Cytol. 1987;31(2):119–24.

Davidson B, Dong HP, Holth A, Berner A, Risberg B. Flow cytometric immunophenotyping of cancer cells in effusion specimens: diagnostic and research applications. Diagn Cytopathol. 2007;35(9):568–78.

Guzman J, Bross KJ, Würtemberger G, Freudenberg N, Costabel U. Tuberculous pleural effusions: lymphocyte phenotypes in comparison with other lymphocyte-rich effusions. Diagn Cytopathol. 1989;5(2): 139–44.

Iqbal J, Liu T, Mapow B, Swami VK, Hou JS. Importance of flow cytometric analysis of serous effusions in the diagnosis of hematopoietic neoplasms in patients with prior hematopoietic malignancies. Anal Quant Cytol Histol. 2010;32(3):161–5.

Kishimoto K, Kitamura T, Hirayama Y, Tate G, Mitsuya T. Cytologic and immunocytochemical features of EBV negative primary effusion lymphoma: report on seven Japanese cases. Diagn Cytopathol. 2009;37(4):293–8.

Mihaescu A, Gebhard S, Chaubert P, Rochat MC, Braunschweig R, Bosman FT, Delacrétaz F, Benhattar J. Application of molecular genetics to the diagnosis of lymphoid-rich effusions: study of 95 cases with concomitant immunophenotyping. Diagn Cytopathol. 2002;27(2):90–5.

Ohori NP, Whisnant RE, Nalesnik MA, Swerdlow SH. Primary pleural effusion posttransplant lymphoproliferative disorder: distinction from secondary involvement and effusion lymphoma. Diagn Cytopathol. 2001;25(1):50–3.

Sasser RL, Yam LT, Li CY. Myeloma with involvement of the serous cavities. Cytologic and immunochemical diagnosis and literature review. Acta Cytol. 1990;34(4):479–85.

Stonesifer KJ, Xiang JH, Wilkinson EJ, Benson NA, Braylan RC. Flow cytometric analysis and cytopathology of body cavity fluids. Acta Cytol. 1987;31(2):125–30.

9
Benign Inflammatory and Other Uncommon Conditions

A number of benign conditions may be routinely encountered in SCFs. A careful evaluation of the various cytologic components in the fluid may suggest a more specific pathologic condition.

- Benign conditions
  - Reactive mesothelial hyperplasia
  - Significance of background cellular composition
- Predominantly blood
- Predominantly lymphocytes
- Predominantly eosinophils
- Predominantly PMNs
- Benign diseases with specific cellular patterns

Benign Diseases with Specific Cellular Patterns (Figs. 9.1, 9.2, 9.3, 9.4, 9.5, 9.6, 9.7, 9.8, 9.9, 9.10, 9.11, 9.12, 9.13, 9.14, 9.15, 9.16 and 9.17)

S.Z. Ali and E.S. Cibas, *Serous Cavity Fluid and Cerebrospinal Fluid Cytopathology*, Essentials in Cytopathology 10, DOI 10.1007/ 978-1-4614-1776-7_9,
© Springer Science+Business Media, LLC 2012

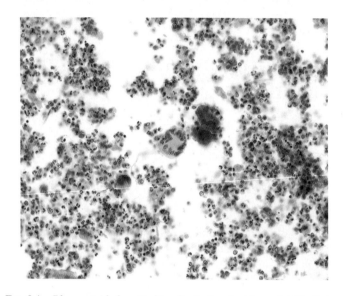

FIG. 9.1. *Rheumatoid pleuritis.* Despite the low incidence (~1%) of pleural effusions caused by systemic diseases, more often connective tissue diseases, such as rheumatoid arthritis or systemic lupus erythematosus, may present with this picture. In this case, SCF with marked acute inflammation and a characteristic multinucleated giant cell (*middle of the field*) juxtaposed with amorphous globular necrotic debris is observed. Bilateral pleural effusions are infrequent in rheumatoid pleuritis, and massive pleural effusions are rare (Papanicolaou, low power).

- Infectious diseases
- Viral, fungal, or parasitic (identify the microorganisms or characteristic associated cellular changes)
- Rheumatoid pleuritis
- Multinucleated giant cells, fibroblasts, and histiocytes in a granular background
- Systemic lupus erythematosus (SLE)
- LE cells in an acute inflammatory background

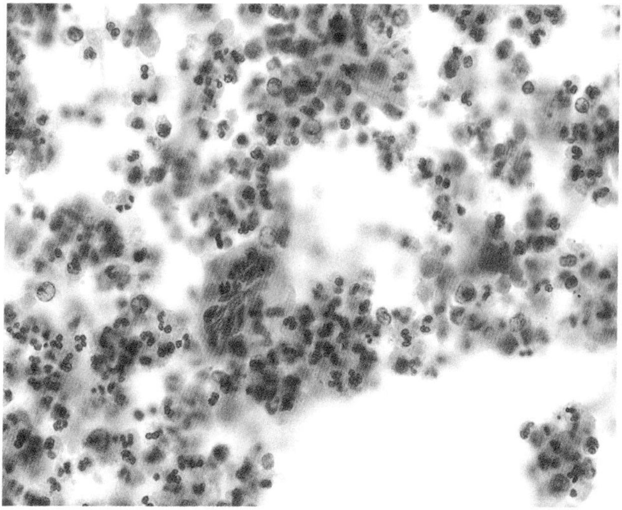

FIG. 9.2. *Rheumatoid pleuritis.* SCF with abundant PMNs and necrotic cellular debris also shows a multinucleated giant histiocyte containing slender elongated and grooved nuclei. These features often constitute the diagnostic triad of rheumatoid pleural effusion: elongated macrophages, giant multinucleated macrophages, and background of granular necrotic debris (Papanicolaou, high power).

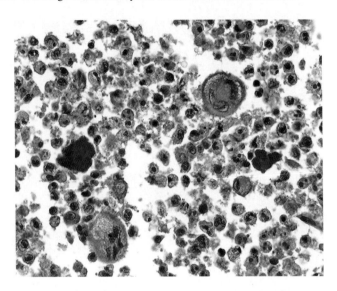

FIG. 9.3. *Rheumatoid pleuritis.* Cell block section from the same case displays multinucleated giant histiocytes, extensive acute inflammation, cellular necrosis, and fragments of amorphous eosinophilic material. Rheumatoid pleuritis characteristically occurs in middle-aged men and can often occur before the onset of the arthritis. Although the absolute incidence of rheumatoid pleural effusion is low, they are one of the more common pulmonary manifestations of rheumatoid arthritis (H & E, high power).

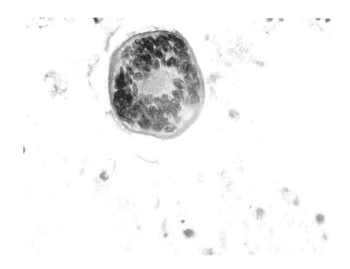

Fig. 9.4. *Rheumatoid pleuritis.* The characteristic multinucleated giant histiocyte from a cell block section is depicted here. The pleural fluid in this disease is exudative, frequently turbid, and may appear milky on gross examination. The fluid shows a characteristic low glucose level. The rheumatoid effusion also has a characteristically low pH, typically between 7.00 and 7.13. The combination of a polymorphonuclear exudate along with a low pleural fluid glucose and pH makes the distinction between rheumatoid effusions and empyema difficult. Hence, a routine cytologic analysis of the effusion is imperative to look for the diagnostic triad (H & E, high power) (Image courtesy of Dr. Y. Erozan).

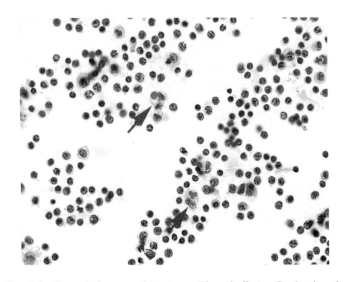

FIG. 9.5. *Systemic lupus erythematosus. Pleural effusion.* Predominantly lymphomononuclear cells with few containing glassy-appearing intracytoplasmic inclusions characteristic of the so-called LE cell (*arrows*). LE cells are leukocytic phagocytes containing hematoxylin bodies representing partially digested lymphocytic nuclei. Pleuropulmonary manifestations in SLE are present in almost half of the patients during the disease course and may be the presenting symptoms in 4–5% of patients. Pleuritis with or without pleural effusion is the most common manifestation and can be particularly troublesome to manage but is rarely life-threatening. Local measures such as talc pleurodesis are often employed if systemic measures fail or when pleural effusion is the only manifestation of lupus (Papanicolaou, low power).

Fig. 9.6. *Systemic lupus erythematosus. Pleural effusion.* Lymphomono-nuclear cells with the characteristic intracytoplasmic bodies "LE" cells. Extremely rarely, systemic lupus erythematosus may present with massive bilateral pleural effusions as the first manifestation months before the patient develops the full-blown syndrome. Studies have shown that the pleural effusion ANA at a titer of [3]1:160 is a sensitive and specific diagnostic biomarker for lupus pleuritis in patients with lupus. However, pleural effusion ANA can occasionally be found in other conditions (Papanicolaou, high power).

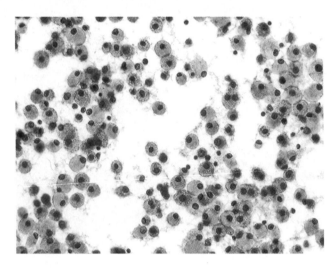

FIG. 9.7. *Chylous effusion*. This ascitic fluid contains an almost pure population of macrophages with characteristic vacuolated "bubbly" cytoplasm indicative of high lipid content. The main clinical manifestations of chylous effusion include dyspnea, edema, abdominal distention, and loss of weight. Common etiologic factors are abdominal injury or surgery, mediastinal irradiation, filariasis, thrombosis of subclavian vein and superior vena cava, malignancies, infections (chest tuberculosis), lymphatic disorders, or idiopathic or drug-associated lymphadenopathy (Papanicolaou, low power).

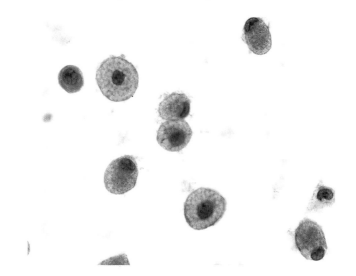

FIG. 9.8. *Chylous effusion.* Chyle is a fluid rich in triglycerides and is characterized by the presence of chylomicrons. This pleural fluid contained numerous large histiocytes with "soap bubble" cytoplasm. Grossly, this effusion had an opaque pale yellow appearance. Other tests for a positive identification of chylous effusion are by Sudan III staining, high triglyceride levels (>1.25 mmol/L), lymphangiography, or lymphangioscintigraphy. Medical thoracoscopic talc pleurodesis, which has an acceptable complication rate and a 100% success rate in the prevention of recurrences, is often considered the standard management approach (Papanicolaou, high power).

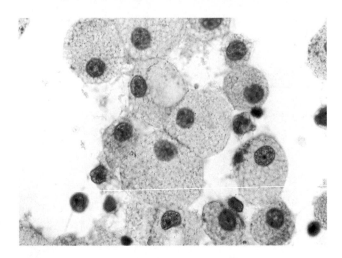

FIG. 9.9. *Chylous effusion*. Numerous macrophages displaying distended and distinctly vacuolated cytoplasm are depicted. These should not be confused with metastatic clear cell neoplasms such as renal cell carcinoma. Chylous ascites is a rare condition. Its etiological factors can be broadly classified as congenital, infective, neoplastic, and traumatic or postsurgical. The combination of chyloperitoneum and chylothorax is even rarer. When abdominal lymphatics are obstructed, chylous ascites results and eventually leads to a chylothorax. The patient typically presents with progressive abdominal distention and weight gain (Papanicolaou, high power).

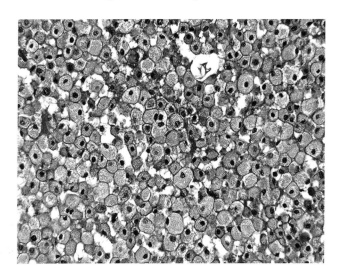

FIG. 9.10. *Chylous effusion.* Cell block section convincingly shows innumerable histiocytes with well-defined cytoplasmic borders containing voluminous amounts of finely vacuolated cytoplasm. Only rare mesothelial cells are seen in such cases (H & E, low power).

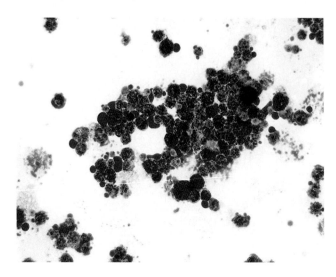

FIG. 9.11. *Chylous effusion.* Oil Red O stain confirms the presence of abundant intracytoplasmic lipid. Treatment modalities for chylous effusion include dietary modification, management of underlying causes, and subcutaneous octreotide. Refractory cases need either open or laparoscopic ligation of the leaking lymphatic channels (low power).

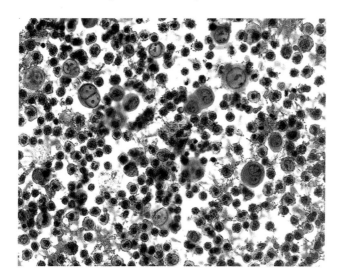

FIG. 9.12. *Varicella-zoster infection.* Pleural effusion in a patient with disseminated VZ infection. Numerous PMNs and few mesothelial cells with totally effaced "ground glass" chromatin containing eosinophilic inclusions (Papanicolaou, high power).

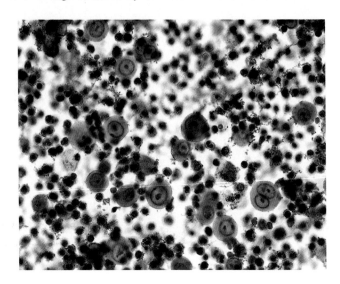

FIG. 9.13. *Varicella-zoster infection.* Notice the characteristic "ground glass" nuclei of the mesothelial cells. A VZV immunoperoxidase stain can also be performed to confirm the diagnosis (Papanicolaou, high power).

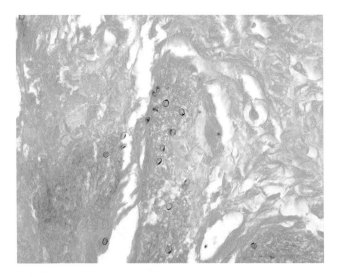

FIG. 9.14. *Pneumocystis jiroveci infection. Pleural effusion.* A silver stain (*GMS*) illustrates the characteristic disk-shaped organisms embedded in a thick proteinaceous precipitate (high power).

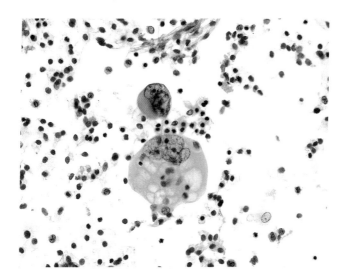

FIG. 9.15. *Radiation changes.* Depicted is a pleural effusion in a patient who received radiation to the chest wall. Bizarre cells with multinucleation and cytoplasmic vacuolization are likely reactive mesothelial cells (Papanicolaou, high power).

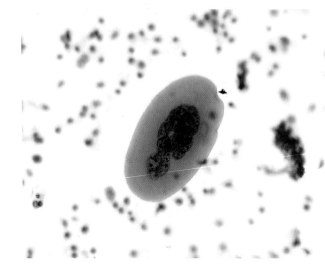

FIG. 9.16. *Radiation changes.* A large mesothelial cell with unusual appearance is seen here. There is multinucleation and a distinct opacity of the cell cytoplasm. This patient had an ovarian adenocarcinoma (Papanicolaou, high power).

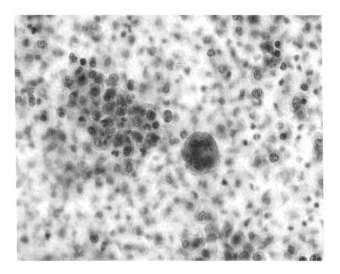

FIG. 9.17. *Extramedullary hematopoiesis.* Ascitic fluid displays mononuclear cells consistent with maturing hematopoietic cells. The large multinucleated cell represents a megakaryocyte (Papanicolaou, high power).

Significance of Background Cellular Composition

- Predominantly blood
  - Traumatic tap
  - Infarct
  - Malignancy
  - Endometriosis

- Predominantly lymphocytes
  - Tuberculosis
  - Malignancy
    - Malignant lymphoma
    - Other malignant neoplasms
- Predominantly eosinophils
  - No specific disease
  - Postpneumothorax
  - Tuberculosis
- Predominantly PMNs
  - Acute inflammatory conditions (e.g., empyema, purulent peritonitis)
  - SLE
- Predominantly anthracotic pigment/carbon-laden macrophages

  - Crack (freebase cocaine) users

Pulmonary Infarct

- A notorious cause of marked mesothelial atypia in pleural fluid
- Single mesothelial cells and fragments (when accompanied by reactive hyperplasia)
- High N/C ratios, prominent nucleoli

Pleural Effusions in HIV-Positive Patients

- General incidence – 7%
- Concomitant pulmonary disease – 96%
  - Bacterial pneumonia
  - Mycobacterial infection
  - Non-Hodgkin's lymphoma
  - Kaposi's sarcoma

Pleural Effusions with Specific Infectious Etiology

- Pneumocystis jiroveci
- CMV
- Varicella zoster
- Microfilaria
- Blastomycosis

Tuberculous Pleuritis/Peritonitis

- Abundant mature-appearing lymphocytes, predominantly CD3 positive on immunostaining
- Macrophages
- Rare mesothelial cells
- Intact granulomas rarely seen

Rheumatoid Pleuritis/Ascites

- Necrotizing granulomatous pleuritis
- Typically large exudative pleural effusions
- Afflicts more men than women and 95% of the patients have high titers of rheumatoid factor (RF)
- In 46% of cases, rheumatoid pleural effusion is diagnosed in close temporal relationship with the diagnosis of RA
- Slender, elongated multinucleated macrophages
- Round giant multinucleated macrophages
- Loosely cohesive fragments of small cytologically bland epithelioid cells
- Pleural effusion with predominant eosinophilia is rare
- Necrotic and amorphous (eosinophilic) background material
- Cell block sections may display fibroconnective tissue fragments lined by hyperplastic mesothelium with squamous metaplasia

Systemic Lupus Erythematosus (SLE)

- Chronic inflammatory autoimmune disorder that predominantly affects women and may affect any organ system
- Serosal cavities often involved with acute recurrent serositis
- Signs and symptoms of lupus pleuritis are nonspecific
- Predominance of PMNs
- LE cells
- Immunological workup typically shows positive response of ANA-speckle, anti-dsDNA, and anti-ENA in patient serum and SCF. High pleural fluid ANA titer (greater than or equal to 1:160) and a PF/S ANA ratio of greater than or equal to 1

Selected Reading

Armbruster C, Schalleschak J, Vetter N, Pokieser L. Pleural effusions in human immunodeficiency virus-infected patients. Correlation with concomitant pulmonary diseases. Acta Cytol. 1995;39(4):698–700.

Dodge JL, Ali SZ. Chylous effusions. Acta Cytol. 2002;46(3):614–6.

Fentanes de Torres E, Guevara E. Pleuritis by radiation: reports of two cases. Acta Cytol. 1981;25(4):427–9.

García-Riego A, Cuiñas C, Vilanova JJ, Ibarrola R. Extramedullary hematopoietic effusions. Acta Cytol. 1998;42(5):1116–20.

Guzman J, Bross KJ, Würtemberger G, Freudenberg N, Costabel U. Tuberculous pleural effusions: lymphocyte phenotypes in comparison with other lymphocyte-rich effusions. Diagn Cytopathol. 1989;5(2):139–44.

Kren L, Rotterova P, Hermanova M, Krenova Z, Sterba J, Dvorak K, Goncharuk V, Wilner GD, McKenna BJ. Chylothorax as a possible diagnostic pitfall: a report of 2 cases with cytologic findings. Acta Cytol. 2005;49(4):441–4.

Matthai SM, Kini U. Diagnostic value of eosinophils in pleural effusion: a prospective study of 26 cases. Diagn Cytopathol. 2003;28(2):96–9.

Naylor B. The pathognomonic cytologic picture of rheumatoid pleuritis. The 1989 Maurice Goldblatt cytology award lecture. Acta Cytol. 1990;34(4):465–73.

Nosanchuk JS, Naylor B. A unique cytologic picture in pleural fluid from patients with rheumatoid arthritis. Am J Clin Pathol. 1968;50(3): 330–5.

Reda MG, Baigelman W. Pleural effusion in systemic lupus erythematosus. Acta Cytol. 1980;24(6):553–7.

Spieler P. The cytologic diagnosis of tuberculosis in pleural effusions. Acta Cytol. 1979;23(5):374–9.

Wojno KJ, Olson JL, Sherman ME. Cytopathology of pleural effusions after radiotherapy. Acta Cytol. 1994;38(1):1–8.

10
Cerebrospinal Fluid

The lumbar puncture (spinal tap) was introduced in 1891, and in 1904 a French neurologist first described malignant cells in cerebrospinal fluid (CSF). Since then, preparatory methods have been refined and diagnostic features described in a number of monographs and atlases, attesting to the importance of CSF cytology for excluding leptomeningeal metastasis in a patient with neurologic symptoms.

Anatomy and Physiology

The brain contains four cavities known as *ventricles*, which communicate with each other and with the subarachnoid space surrounding the brain and spinal cord. The ventricles are lined by a cuboidal ciliated cell layer called the *ependyma*. In some areas, the ependyma differentiates into a complex villous structure called the *choroid plexus,* which is composed of a single layer of cuboidal nonciliated cells overlying a vascular core. The choroid plexus produces most of the CSF by both filtering plasma across capillary walls and actively secreting fluid. After leaving the ventricles via the midline foramen of Magendie and the two lateral foramina of Luschka, CSF circulates in the *subarachnoid space*, formed by the *leptomeninges* (composed of the pia mater and arachnoid mater),

S.Z. Ali and E.S. Cibas, *Serous Cavity Fluid and Cerebrospinal Fluid Cytopathology*, Essentials in Cytopathology 10, DOI 10.1007/978-1-4614-1776-7_10, © Springer Science+Business Media, LLC 2012

over cerebral and spinal surfaces. Fluid is then reabsorbed by the arachnoid granulations into the venous system, and the cycle begins anew.

The total volume of CSF in the adult is about 150 mL. Approximately 500 mL/day is produced (0.35 mL/min), meaning that the CSF is renewed three or four times daily.

Obtaining and Preparing the Specimen

Most CSF specimens are obtained by lumbar puncture (LP), in which a needle is passed through the intervertebral space at L3–L4 or L4–L5. Rarely, because of inflammation at these sites or a bony abnormality, the specimen must be obtained from the cisterna magna at the base of the brain. Cisternal CSF sometimes yields positive results when LP is negative. CSF is sometimes aspirated directly from a lateral ventricle during a neurosurgical procedure; such specimens often contain fragments of normal brain. In patients undergoing chemotherapy for leptomeningeal metastases, a silicone pouch (Ommaya reservoir) is implanted in subcutaneous tissue, and a cannula leads from the pouch into a lateral ventricle through a 3-mm burr hole. This is an efficient way to introduce chemotherapeutic drugs and to withdraw CSF periodically for examination.

A minimum of 1 mL should be collected for cytologic evaluation, but 3 mL or more is preferable, and at least 10 mL is considered ideal. Surprisingly, the amount of CSF removed does not affect the likelihood that a patient will develop a headache.

Fluid should be collected fresh and delivered to the laboratory as quickly as possible to prevent cellular deterioration. If the specimen cannot be prepared immediately, it should be refrigerated at 4°C. If a delay of more than 48 h is anticipated, the sample can be preserved by adding an equal volume of 50% ethanol. A CSF sample for cytologic examination should never be frozen.

The most common ways to prepare specimens are by cytocentrifugation, membrane filtration, and thin-layer preparation. Because greater technical skill is needed to process membrane filtration specimens, this is best done in a laboratory that specializes in this method. Cytocentrifugation has greater flexibility, because both alcohol-fixed and air-dried slides can be prepared using this method. Lymphoid cells are best evaluated using air-dried preparations; thus it is advisable to prepare both alcohol-fixed Papanicolaou-stained slides and air-dried Wright-stained slides. Depending on the volume and cellularity of the specimen, additional slides can be used for immunocytochemical studies if needed.

Blood is a common contaminant. The needle lacerates the veins that course along the crowded nerve roots of the cauda equina in 75% of LPs, and this can create diagnostic problems. Neutrophils, if accompanied by red blood cells, should not necessarily be interpreted as evidence of acute meningitis. Similarly, leukemic blasts from peripheral blood can contaminate the fluid, leading to an erroneous impression of meningeal involvement by leukemia. It takes only a minute amount of blood to alter the cellular composition of CSF significantly, an amount that can be invisible to the naked eye. Because alcohol fixation lyses red blood cells, contamination is best detected on air-dried preparations. If red blood cells are present, the possibility of contamination by peripheral blood blasts should be raised.

Reporting Terminology

As with most cytologic specimens, CSF cytology results are commonly reported as either "negative for malignancy," "atypical," "suspicious," or "positive." Over 90% of CSF specimens are assigned a cytologic diagnosis of "negative for malignant cells." Many show only a small number of lymphocytes and monocytes, essentially a normal CSF.

The primary role of CSF cytology is to exclude circulating malignant cells in CSF pathways. Although a specific diagnosis of some benign diseases (e.g., cryptococcosis) can be made cytologically, in most nonmalignant CNS diseases, CSF cytology is frustratingly unrevealing. The myriad diseases that cause aseptic meningitis, for example, have as their final common denominator nothing more than a lymphocytic and/or monocytic pleocytosis. The cause is identified by other clinical and laboratory methods.

Accuracy

The sensitivity of CSF cytology for detecting malignant cells is about 60%. But sensitivity depends on several factors. First and foremost, a positive CSF sample will occur only if a CNS malignancy actually invades into a ventricle or the subarachnoid space.

The sensitivity of CSF cytology depends upon:

- The number of specimens examined
- The volume of fluid submitted
- The extent of leptomeningeal disease
- The site from which the sample was obtained (lumbar vs. cisterna magna)

The sensitivity of a single cytologic examination is 54% but increases to 84% with a second sample. Smaller incremental increases in sensitivity are observed with more than two specimens. Sensitivity is dependent of sample volume: sensitivity is greater if 10 mL is submitted rather than 3 mL. Sensitivity also depends on the extent of leptomeningeal disease: 38% for focal and 66% for disseminated leptomeningeal tumor. Similarly, only 50% of patients with early meningeal involvement by acute lymphoblastic leukemia have a suspicious or positive CSF. The site from which the sample is obtained can also affect the sensitivity: if LP specimens are negative, a tap from the cisterna magna sometimes yields malignant cells.

The specificity of CSF cytology is high. False-positive diagnoses are estimated at 2–3%. The most common cause is the overdiagnosis of lymphoma or leukemia, particularly in patients with herpes zoster meningitis, cryptococcal meningitis, Lyme disease, viral meningitis, and in LP specimens contaminated with blood.

In light of these data, the American College of Physicians has determined that cytologic examination of CSF for meningeal malignancy has moderate sensitivity and high specificity.

Normal Elements

Normal CSF is sparsely cellular and, in adults, contains less than five cells/mm^3 (equivalent to 5,000 cells/mL). In newborns the fluid is more cellular.

Normal CSF elements:

- Common

  - Lymphocytes
  - Monocytes

- Rare

  - Choroid plexus/ependymal cells
  - Brain fragments
  - Germinal matrix
  - Chondrocytes
  - Bone marrow

Normal CSF is composed of lymphocytes and monocytes (Figs. 10.1 and 10.2). Only small numbers of mature lymphocytes are present in normal CSF, but their number can increase markedly, particularly in viral meningitis and other inflammatory or infectious conditions. Such specimens can be highly cellular, with a minor population of so-called atypical lymphoid cells that are large and may show irregular nuclear contours, with clefting, blebs, and nucleoli.

Monocytes are also present in normal CSF. Larger than lymphocytes, they have folded, kidney bean-shaped nuclei and a moderate amount of cytoplasm.

Choroid plexus and ependymal cells are seen in less than 0.5% of LP specimens. These cells have round to oval, regular nuclei, a moderate amount of cytoplasm, and are seen singly or in small clusters (Fig. 10.3). Brain fragments have a fibrillary texture and contain glial cells, neurons, and capillaries (Fig. 10.4). They are seen in samples taken directly from the ventricles because the needle traverses brain parenchyma, and are not seen in LP samples. Rarely, isolated neurons are present (Fig. 10.5).

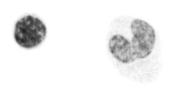

FIG. 10.1. *Normal CSF.* Lymphocytes and monocytes are the usual components of a normal CSF (Papanicolaou-stained cytocentrifuge preparation).

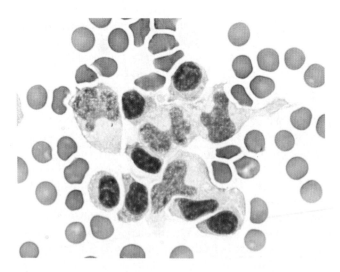

FIG. 10.2. *Normal CSF.* Lymphocytes and monocytes (Wright–Giemsa-stained cytocentrifuge preparation).

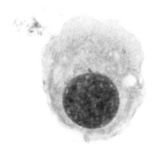

FIG. 10.3. *Choroid plexus/ependymal cells.* These cells are rare in CSF; even when present, their number is usually small. They may be isolated or arranged in small clusters. Note the dispersed chromatin texture of the nucleus and the abundant cytoplasm (Wright–Giemsa stain).

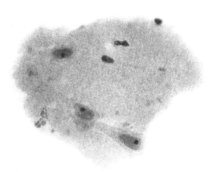

FIG. 10.4. *Brain tissue.* This fragment, obtained from a ventricular tap, has a fibrillary texture and contains normal glial cells and neurons. Some fragments may contain capillaries (Papanicolaou stain).

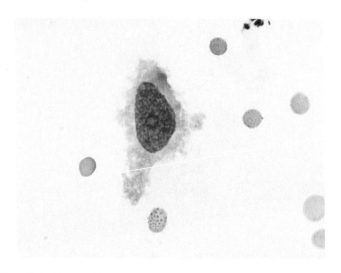

FIG. 10.5. *Neuron.* Neurons have an angular cell shape, a round nucleus, and a prominent nucleolus (Wright–Giemsa stain).

In CSF from neonates, most commonly those born prematurely, one occasionally sees small, immature cells of germinal matrix origin. Germinal matrix cells lie beneath the ependyma in the wall of the lateral ventricles and exfoliate when there is subependymal and intraventricular hemorrhage (Fig. 10.6). They are often clustered and molded to one another, thus mimicking a small cell malignancy (see section "Medulloblastoma" below). Because of their frequent association with hemorrhage, these cells are often accompanied by hemosiderin-laden macrophages.

If the LP needle is inserted too far anteriorly, the CSF can be contaminated by chondrocytes (Fig. 10.7) or bone marrow cells (Fig. 10.8) from the intervertebral disk or vertebral body, respectively. These cells, seen in less than 1% of CSF specimens, should not be mistaken for malignant cells. Other common contaminants are starch granules and squamous cells. Although mitoses are more common in malignant specimens, they are occasionally seen in benign conditions such as bacterial and viral meningitis.

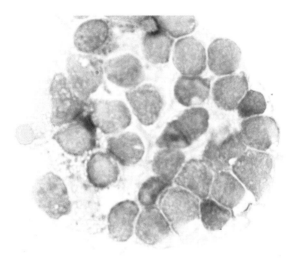

Fɪɢ. 10.6. *Germinal matrix.* Clusters of small cells accompanied by macrophages are seen in CSF (Wright–Giemsa stain).

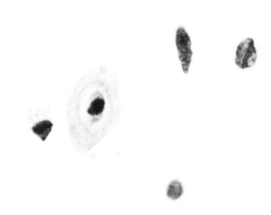

Fɪɢ. 10.7. *Chondrocyte.* Rarely seen in CSF, chondrocytes are large cells with a pyknotic nucleus surrounded by an extracellular mucopolysaccharide matrix that stains blue purple with the Papanicolaou stain (Papanicolaou stain).

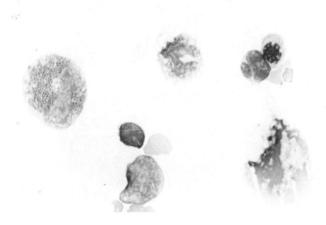

Fɪɢ. 10.8. *Bone marrow.* If the needle penetrates a vertebral body, immature erythroid and myeloid elements from normal bone marrow are sam-
pled, as seen here (Wright–Giemsa stain).

Abnormal Inflammatory Cells

Inflammatory cells such as macrophages, plasma cells, and eosinophils are an abnormal finding in CSF. They may accompany malignancy, but are also seen in a variety of nonneoplastic conditions.

Macrophages have abundant, vacuolated cytoplasm that sometimes contains ingested cells, organisms, or pigment.

Macrophages in CSF are associated with:

- Meningitis
- Subarachnoid hemorrhage
- Intraventricular hemorrhage
- Cerebral infarction
- Posttreatment inflammation
- Multiple sclerosis

Plasma cells are also an abnormal but nonspecific finding in CSF.

Plasma cells in CSF are associated with:

- Viral meningitis (e.g., enterovirus, HIV)
- Lyme disease
- Tuberculosis
- Cysticercosis
- Syphilis
- Multiple sclerosis

Polymorphonuclear leukocytes are a normal finding if there is contamination by peripheral blood, but numerous neutrophils unaccompanied by a proportionate increase in red blood cells raise the possibility of acute meningitis (Fig. 10.9). In a patient with AIDS, numerous neutrophils are highly suggestive of cytomegalovirus (CMV) radiculopathy. Viral cytopathic inclusions, however, are not seen. The diagnosis of CMV radiculopathy can be confirmed by viral culture.

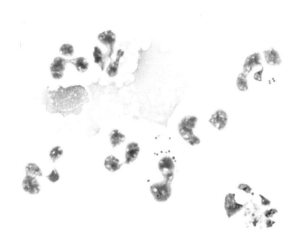

Fig. 10.9. *Acute bacterial (pneumococcal) meningitis.* There are numerous neutrophils and bacteria (Wright–Giemsa stain).

Differential diagnosis – neutrophils in CSF:

- Peripheral blood contamination
- Acute bacterial meningitis
- CMV radiculopathy
- Toxoplasma meningoencephalitis
- Viral meningitis (early stage)

Eosinophils are rare in CSF; when present, especially in large numbers, they suggest a parasitic infection, particularly *Taenia solium* (see section "Cysticercosis" below) and *Angiostrongylus cantonensis* (see section "Angiostrongyliasis" below).

Differential diagnosis – eosinophils in CSF:

- Parasites
- *Coccidioides immitis*
- Ventriculoperitoneal shunts
- Rocky Mountain spotted fever

Nonneoplastic Disorders

Acute Bacterial Meningitis

Many bacteria can cause meningitis, including *Neisseria meningitidis* (meningococcus), *Haemophilus influenzae*, *Streptococcus pneumoniae* (pneumococcus) (Fig. 10.9), and *Listeria monocytogenes*.

Cytomorphology of acute bacterial meningitis:

- Numerous neutrophils
- Bacteria (may or may not be seen)

Because bacterial meningitis can be fatal if not treated immediately, prompt diagnosis is crucial. Any CSF sample composed predominantly of neutrophils should be considered high probability for bacterial meningitis; precise identification of the organism depends on microbiologic cultures.

> Differential diagnosis of acute bacterial meningitis:
>
> - Traumatic tap
> - Toxoplasma meningoencephalitis
> - CMV radiculopathy
> - Aseptic meningitis (early)

Neutrophils admixed with red blood cells and other blood elements are a normal finding resulting from a traumatic tap. Abundant neutrophils are seen in other conditions, such as toxoplasmosis (see below), CMV radiculopathy, and in the early stages of aseptic meningitis.

Aseptic Meningitis

Aseptic meningitis is a misnomer, but the term is ingrained in clinical practice. Despite its name, it is most commonly caused by an infectious organism, usually a virus. The clinical course is less fulminant than that of acute bacterial (pyogenic) meningitis. Aseptic meningitis is usually self-limited and is treated symptomatically. The most common pathogen is one of the enteroviruses (non-paralytic poliovirus, echovirus, and coxsackieviruses).

> Cytomorphology of aseptic meningitis:
>
> - Increase in lymphocytes and monocytes
> - Small proportion of "atypical" lymphocytes

The cytologic findings are nonspecific. There is an increased number of predominantly small, mature lymphocytes, but also monocytes, plasma cells, and enlarged (so-called atypical) lymphocytes, some of which have prominent nucleoli and irregular nuclear contours (Fig. 10.10). In the early stages, neutrophils are present. Viral inclusions are rarely seen in CSF.

Aseptic meningitis is caused by a wide range of organisms, systemic diseases, and miscellaneous conditions (Table 10.1), with identical cytologic findings. It is seen in about 10% of patients within 1–2 weeks of seroconversion due to HIV-1. Aseptic meningitis occurs in some patients with Lyme disease.

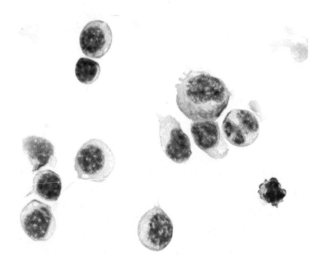

FIG. 10.10. *Aseptic meningitis (viral)*. An increased number of lymphocytes are present, including occasional so-called atypical lymphoid cells: larger cells with larger nuclei, some of which have irregular contours, more finely dispersed chromatin, and prominent nucleoli (Wright–Giemsa stain).

TABLE 10.1. Partial list of causes of aseptic meningitis.

- Viruses
  - Enteroviruses
  - HIV
  - Herpes simplex virus (Mollaret's meningitis)
  - Varicella zoster virus
  - Mumps
  - Arboviruses
  - Arenavirus (lymphocytic choriomeningitis)
- Bacteria
  - *Borrelia burgdorferi* (Lyme disease)
  - *Treponema pallidum* (syphilis)
  - *Mycobacterium tuberculosis*
  - Ehrlichiosis
  - *Mycoplasma pneumoniae*

(continued)

TABLE 10.1. (continued)

- Fungi
  - *Cryptococcus neoformans*
  - *Histoplasma capsulatum*
  - *Coccidioides immitis*
- Systemic diseases
  - Behçet's disease
  - Sarcoidosis
- Other
  - Drugs
  - Vaccines
  - Parainfectious syndrome (acute disseminated encephalomyelitis)
  - Vasculitis

A rare form of aseptic meningitis, *idiopathic recurrent meningitis*, also known as *Mollaret's meningitis* (MM) after the man who first described the disease in 1944, is characterized by recurring attacks of fever, headache, and neck stiffness. Symptoms appear suddenly, last for 5–7 days, resolve spontaneously, but recur days or years later. Herpes simplex viruses 1 and 2 have been identified as putative causative agents in some cases. The diagnosis of MM is made clinically after excluding other causes of aseptic meningitis. Cytologic findings are nonspecific, but there is often a marked predominance of monocytes. So-called Mollaret cells, monocytes with deep nuclear clefts that impart a footprint-like appearance to the nucleus, are seen within the first 24 h of the onset of symptoms. They are characteristic of but not specific for MM; they can be seen in other diseases like sarcoidosis and Behçet's disease.

Differential diagnosis of aseptic meningitis:

- Primary CNS lymphoma
- Secondary involvement by lymphoma
- Acute leukemia

A polymorphous lymphoid population supports the diagnosis of a benign, reactive process. Nevertheless, the presence of some "atypical" lymphocytes raises the possibility of malignant lymphoma. Some lymphomas in the CNS are accompanied by numerous small, reactive T lymphocytes and can, in fact, mimic aseptic meningitis. Because the cells in most cases of aseptic meningitis are T cells, immunocytochemistry and flow cytometry are useful in selected cases. If all the lymphoid cells are T cells, a malignant lymphoma is unlikely, because most lymphomas, including primary CNS lymphomas, are B-cell neoplasms.

In contrast to viral meningitis, the meningeal infiltrate in Lyme disease is comprised of B-cells. In order to distinguish the florid pleocytosis in some cases of Lyme disease from lymphoma, demonstration of polyclonal vs. monoclonal expression of kappa and lambda light chains is necessary.

Cryptococcal Meningitis

The only organism that is identified cytologically with any frequency in CSF is *Cryptococcus neoformans*, which causes disease in both healthy and immunocompromised persons.

Cytomorphology of cryptococcal meningitis:

- Round yeast forms
- Variable size: 5–15 μm diameter
- Pink/purple (Papanicolaou stain)
- Asymmetric, narrow-based budding
- Mucin-positive capsule
- Refractile artifact

The degree of inflammation is variable. There can be a marked lymphocytic/monocytic pleocytosis, in which case organisms are hard to identify. Alternatively, there may be abundant organisms and very little inflammatory response (Fig. 10.11). *C. neoformans* is sometimes perfectly round, but often indented. The indentations trap air under the coverslip, resulting in a crystal-like refractile artifact.

Toxoplasmosis

In immunocompromised patients, the protozoon *Toxoplasma gondii* can cause a variety of diseases of the CNS, including meningoencephalitis.

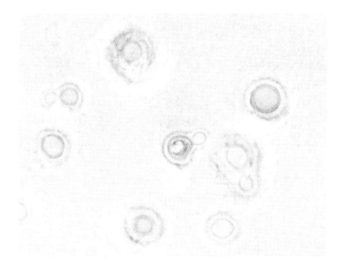

FIG. 10.11. *Cryptococcal meningitis.* The organisms have a mucopoly-saccharide capsule. Note the characteristic thin-necked budding (Papani-colaou stain).

Cytomorphology of Toxoplasma meningoencephalitis:

- Neutrophils
- Mononuclear cells
- Tachyzoites

Toxoplasma tachyzoites are small, crescent-shaped organisms, 3–6 μm in length, with a tiny, round nucleus. In patients who develop obstructive hydrocephalus, tachyzoites are more likely to be found in ventricular rather than lumbar samples.

Cysticercosis

Cerebral cysticercosis results from colonization of the brain by larvae of the tapeworm *Taenia solium*. Clinical symptoms are nonspecific. Imaging studies usually show a focal lesion in the brain.

Cytomorphology of cysticercosis:

- Eosinophils (2–70% of cells)
- Mononuclear cells

Larvae are not seen in the CSF. Serologic tests confirm the diagnosis.

Angiostrongyliasis

The lungworm *Angiostrongylus cantonensis* is endemic to Asia, particularly the Pacific region, but is found elsewhere. Infection, with subsequent migration of larvae to the CNS, results in eosinophilic meningitis. Headache is the most common presenting symptom. The percentage of eosinophils in CSF is usually very high (20–70%). Larvae are occasionally seen in the fluid. Focal lesions on computed tomography examination are usually absent, thus helping to distinguish angiostrongyliasis from cysticercosis. The disease is usually self-limited, and patients recover completely.

Other roundworm infections that usually present as eosinophilic meningitis are *Gnathostoma spinigerum*, a parasite of dogs and cats, and *Baylisascaris procyonis*, a parasite of raccoons.

Primary Amebic Meningoencephalitis

The free living ameba *Naegleria fowleri* can cause acute meningoencephalitis. The organisms enter the subarachnoid space through the nose, often while a person is swimming in stagnant water or in an unchlorinated swimming pool. The organisms are best seen on wet preparations, where their motility can be appreciated. With conventional cytologic preparations they can be difficult to distinguish from mononuclear cells. They have a relatively large nucleus and little cytoplasm, unlike *Entamoeba histolytica*. Fortunately, the disease is rare; it can be fatal within several days.

Primary amebic meningoencephalitis must be distinguished from an amebic brain abscess caused by *Entamoeba histolytica*. Amoebae are not seen in the CSF with the latter infection.

Neoplasms

Involvement of the subarachnoid space by malignancy occurs in 5–8% of patients with cancer. Some tumors, like small cell carcinoma of the lung (11%) and melanoma (20%), have a greater predilection than most for involving the leptomeninges. Malignant cells gain access to the subarachnoid space by hematogenous dissemination, direct extension from a parenchymal brain lesion, or by tracking along spinal or cranial nerves. Involvement of the leptomeninges by tumor is often referred to as carcinomatous (or lymphomatous, etc.) meningitis, but the term leptomeningeal metastasis is best because it applies to all tumors that involved the meninges.

The clinical presentation of patients with leptomeningeal metastasis is highly variable. Symptoms can include headache, mental changes, gait difficulty, diplopia, back pain, and lower extremity weakness. Gadolinium-enhanced magnetic resonance imaging often shows suspicious enhancement of the leptomeninges when malignancy is present, but CSF for cytology is needed to confirm the diagnosis.

CSF examination is an important component in the diagnosis of leptomeningeal metastasis. Many patients have elevated opening pressure, with elevated protein and depressed glucose levels. Cytologic examination of CSF, however, is essential for documenting leptomeningeal metastasis. When present, malignant cells are usually easily identified in CSF samples because they are strikingly different from the normal cells of CSF. Thus, most CSF samples are easily classified as either negative or positive for malignancy. When findings are inconclusive, often because of scant cellularity or poor preservation, a "suspicious" or "atypical" interpretation is warranted. Not surprisingly, the greatest difficulty is in the diagnosis of lymphoma and leukemia.

When malignant cells are identified, the clinical history often points to their site of origin. In most cases the patient is known to have a malignancy, and the findings simply confirm metastasis. The most commonly encountered malignancies in CSF are lung and breast cancer, melanoma, lymphoma, and leukemia.

In about 10% of patients with a positive CSF, cytologic examination provides the first documentation of a neoplasm. The lung is by far the most common occult primary site, followed by gastric cancer and melanoma. Patients with lymphoma, leukemia, or a primary CNS tumor can also present with a positive CSF examination. Curiously, a primary breast cancer is very rarely occult when CSF involvement is detected.

Likely primaries in a patient with positive CSF and no history of cancer:

- Lung
- Stomach
- Melanoma
- Lymphoma
- CNS

Metastatic tumors are much more frequent than primary CNS tumors in CSF; primary CNS tumors account for only 6% of all positive CSF samples.

Immunocytochemistry is not needed to diagnose most cases of leptomeningeal metastasis. In selected cases, however, it is useful for establishing a likely primary site, for example, in a patient whose cancer first manifests itself as a positive CSF. Epithelial markers can establish a diagnosis of carcinoma and exclude the possibility of lymphoma, melanoma, and a primary glioma. Glial fibrillary acidic protein (GFAP) differentiates glial from non-glial tissue and can be used to confirm a primary CNS origin for malignant cells in CSF. GFAP is useful in establishing a diagnosis of malignancy when the cytologic examination is equivocal because normal CSF obtained by LP does not contain GFAP-positive cells.

The median survival of untreated patients with leptomeningeal metastasis is 1 month. Treatment stabilizes or improves about 75% of patients, but it is almost always palliative rather than curative, because current treatments cannot eliminate tumor from the subarachnoid space. The median survival of treated patients ranges from 4 to 10 months and depends in part on the tumor type: breast cancer and lymphoma respond better than most other tumors. Radiation therapy is often considered in patients with bulky and/or symptomatic leptomeningeal metastasis and is especially helpful in relieving pain and other symptoms. Intrathecal chemotherapy, administered by Ommaya reservoir, has been the mainstay of treatment for leptomeningeal metastasis, but its palliative effects are usually short-lived. The most commonly used intrathecal agents are methotrexate, cytarabine, and thiotepa. Systemic chemotherapy is gaining acceptance for treating leptomeningeal metastasis because of its greater ability to penetrate bulkier tumor deposits.

Metastatic Solid Tumors

Carcinoma of the Lung

All four of the common histologic subtypes of lung cancer (adenocarcinoma, squamous cell carcinoma, large cell carcinoma, and small cell carcinoma) can metastasize to the CSF pathways. Adenocarcinomas of the lung are common and squamous cell carcinomas uncommon in CSF.

Cytomorphology – adenocarcinoma of the lung (Fig. 10.12):

- Isolated cells and/or small clusters
- Large cells
- Abundant cytoplasm
- Eccentric nucleus

The differential diagnosis of metastatic adenocarcinoma of the lung to CSF includes macrophages, plasma cells, and ependymal/choroid plexus cells. Macrophages have smaller nuclei that are pale and often folded or curved, with granular and microvacuolated cytoplasm (Fig. 10.13). Plasma cells are smaller than the cells of an adenocarcinoma of the lung, with more condensed chromatin and a tell-tale perinuclear hof. Ependymal/choroid plexus cells are rare in CSF; when present, they are few in number, usually with round, centrally placed nuclei.

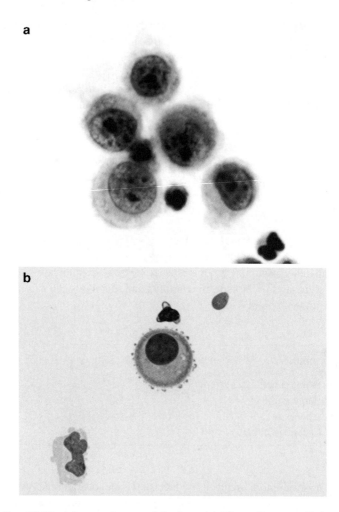

FIG. 10.12. *Adenocarcinoma of the lung.* (**a**) The malignant cells have large, hyperchromatic nuclei and abundant cytoplasm (Papanicolaou stain). (**b**) Note the eccentric placement of the nucleus and the cytoplasmic blebs. A red blood cell, lymphocyte, and monocyte are present for comparison (Wright–Giemsa stain).

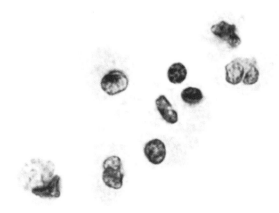

Fɪɢ. 10.13. *Macrophages.* Macrophages have abundant cytoplasm and are seen in benign and malignant conditions (Papanicolaou stain).

Cytomorphology – small cell carcinoma of the lung:

- Isolated cells and/or clustered
- Small cells
- Nuclear molding
- Karyorrhexis
- Mitoses

Small cell carcinomas of the lung appear as small isolated or clustered cells in CSF. When isolated, they are easily mistaken for lymphocytes. Finding clusters with their characteristic molding is often essential for diagnosis (Fig. 10.14). Linear, molded arrangements with a "vertebral body" appearance are seen. The differential diagnosis includes other small cell malignancies, most of them pediatric, like medulloblastoma. A cytomorphologic distinction is impossible, but this rarely presents a problem because patients have a history of small cell carcinoma or a suspicious lung mass.

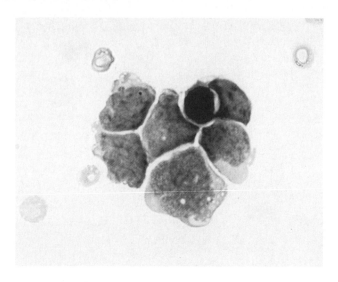

FIG. 10.14. *Small cell carcinoma of the lung.* The small cells have dispersed chromatin, indistinct nucleoli, and scant cytoplasm. Nuclear molding is prominent (Wright–Giemsa stain).

Carcinoma of the Breast

Breast cancer not uncommonly metastasizes to the CSF. In contrast to lung cancer, it is rare that a positive CSF is the presenting finding in a woman with breast cancer.

Cytomorphology – ductal breast cancer (Fig. 10.15):

- Isolated cells or small groups
- Linear rows, rings (rare)
- Large cells
- Round nucleus
- Prominent nucleolus
- Scant cytoplasm (often)

The large cannonball-like arrangements typical of breast cancer cells in pleural fluid are almost never seen in CSF. Instead, the malignant cells are usually dispersed as isolated cells. Nuclei are round or irregular, and some cells can be binucleated.

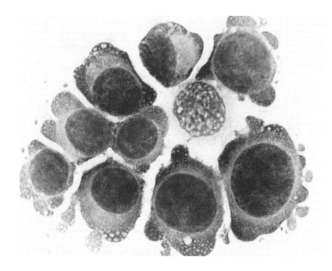

FIG. 10.15. *Ductal carcinoma of the breast.* The malignant cells of this Bloom–Richardson grade 3 ductal cancer are round, large, and highly variable in size. Cytoplasmic blebs are commonly seen (Wright–Giemsa stain).

Cytomorphology – lobular breast cancer:

- Small- to medium-sized cells
- Isolated cells
- Signet-ring shapes

The differential diagnosis of ductal and lobular breast cancers is similar to that for adenocarcinoma of the lung and includes macrophages, and ependymal/choroid plexus cells. Macrophages have smaller, pale, often folded or curved nuclei, with abundant granular and microvacuolated cytoplasm (see Fig. 10.13). Ependymal/choroid plexus cells are rare in CSF; when present, they are few in number and usually have a round, centrally placed nucleus. Some lobular breast cancer cells in CSF form linear arrangements reminiscent of the vertebral body-like structures seen in patients with small cell carcinoma.

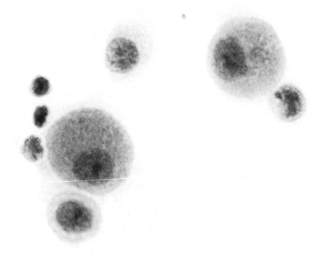

Fig. 10.16. *Melanoma.* Melanoma cells tend to be isolated or only loosely aggregated (Papanicolaou stain).

Melanoma

Melanoma can metastasize to the meninges from a primary in the skin or other site, but it can also (rarely) arise in the leptomeninges as a primary CNS neoplasm. In a condition known as melanosis cerebri, the meninges contain melanocytes; presumably, it is these cells that give rise to leptomeningeal melanomas.

Cytomorphology of melanoma (Fig. 10.16):

- Large cells
- Macronucleolus
- Melanin (not always)
- Melanophages

With a history of melanoma, the diagnosis is straightforward in most cases. Rarely, as in a patient without a documented melanoma whose malignant cells lack visible melanin, the distinction from a carcinoma may require immunocytochemistry. Stains for HMB45 and S-100 are generally positive, whereas stains for keratin and epithelial membrane antigen are negative.

Leukemia

Acute Lymphoblastic Leukemia

Acute lymphoblastic leukemia (ALL), a malignancy of lymphocyte precursors that arises from the bone marrow, is the most common malignancy in children. The peak incidence is between the ages of 2 and 7 years, but adults are also affected. Patients often present with pallor and weakness because of anemia, and bleeding due to thrombocytopenia. They can have lymphadenopathy, hepatosplenomegaly, and an anterior mediastinal mass. The diagnosis is made by bone marrow aspiration and biopsy, which shows replacement of normal elements by lymphoblasts. CNS involvement is present at initial diagnosis in 5% of cases and is usually occult. In fact, 75% of ALL patients with leptomeningeal metastasis are asymptomatic.

The appearance of the blasts is variable. According to the French–American–British (FAB) classification system, ALL is divided into types L1, L2, and L3 based on the cytomorphologic appearance on air-dried Wright–Giemsa-stained preparations (Fig. 10.17). The WHO recommends that the FAB classification be abandoned, because morphological classification has no clinical or prognostic relevance. Instead, the WHO advocates the use of a combined immunophenotypic and cytogenetic classification which carries prognostic significance. Nevertheless, knowledge of the spectrum of morphologic appearances of ALL can be very useful in evaluating CSF, particularly in correlating CSF findings with prior bone marrow aspirates.

Cytomorphology of ALL (Wright–Giemsa-type stains):
- L1

   - Small blasts
   - Round nucleus (rare clefts)
   - Fine chromatin
   - Inconspicuous nucleolus
   - Scant, slightly basophilic cytoplasm

(continued)

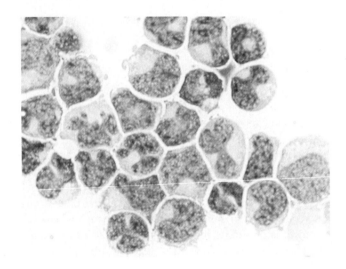

FIG. 10.17. *Acute lymphoblastic leukemia.* Depending on the subtype, the blasts of acute lymphoblastic leukemia may have several different appearances, which are best appreciated on air-dried preparations. L2 blasts (seen here) are larger, with irregular nuclei and more abundant cytoplasm (Wright–Giemsa stain).

- L2
  - Larger blasts
  - Irregular nucleus
  - Fine chromatin
  - Prominent nucleolus
  - Abundant cytoplasm

- L3
  - Coarse chromatin
  - Multiple nucleoli
  - Dark blue cytoplasm
  - Small cytoplasmic vacuoles (lipid)
  - Indistinguishable from Burkitt lymphoma

In a small percentage of cases, the cells of ALL contain azurophilic cytoplasmic inclusions that resemble myeloid granules.

The treatment of ALL in children is one of the great successes of chemotherapy. At one time ALL was almost invariably fatal; today nearly 60% of children are long-term survivors of the disease. CNS prophylaxis is a mainstay of therapy. Without CNS prophylaxis, more than 50% of patients would develop CNS leukemia. Although prophylactic treatment of the CNS with radiotherapy to the cranium and intrathecal methotrexate has reduced the incidence of such relapses dramatically, they still occur in 5–10% of cases. Therefore, periodic monitoring of CSF for the presence of blasts is essential.

Differential diagnosis of ALL:

- Reactive lymphocytes (e.g., aseptic meningitis)
- Peripheral blood contamination

When the sample is hypercellular, the diagnosis is usually straightforward, particularly with air-dried Wright–Giemsa-stained slides, which accentuate the characteristic morphologic features. Sparsely cellular samples can be difficult. Immunocytochemistry for terminal deoxytransferase (Tdt), a nuclear enzyme found in 90–95% of L1 and L2 leukemias (but not in type L3), can be extremely useful in distinguishing blasts from reactive lymphocytes, which are consistently negative for this marker. An aliquot of fluid is also often sent to the hematology laboratory, and blasts, if present, are noted in the differential count. Contamination of CSF by blasts in peripheral blood must be excluded, because this can result in a false-positive diagnosis. If CSF contains leukemic blasts admixed with red blood cells, the specimen is essentially noncontributory. The only exception is a patient in remission, whose peripheral blood counts are negative for blasts. In such a patient, a traumatic tap with blasts is diagnostic of a CSF recurrence.

Acute Myeloid Leukemia

The acute myeloid leukemias (AML) are neoplastic proliferations of the myeloid progenitor cells: immature granulocytes, monocytes, erythrocytes, and megakaryocytes. They are more common in adults than in children. AML can involve CSF either at presentation or subsequently, although CSF involvement is less common than in ALL.

The French–American–British system recognizes eight morphologic types of AML based on bone marrow aspirates:

- AML undifferentiated (M0)
- AML without maturation (M1)
- AML with maturation (M2)
- Acute promyelocytic leukemia (M3)
- Acute myelomonocytic leukemia (M4)
- Acute monocytic leukemia (M5)
- Erythroleukemia (M6)
- Acute megakaryoblastic leukemia (M7)

These subtypes have somewhat different clinical presentations. For example, it is more common for patients with acute myelomonocytic leukemia (AML M4) to have CNS involvement at the time of presentation than for those with other types of AML. As with ALL, the WHO recommends abandoning the FAB classification for AML and replacing it with a system that relies more on clinical and cytogenetic criteria. The WHO subtypes of AML are:

- AML with recurrent cytogenetic abnormalities
- AML with multilineage dysplasia
- AML and myelodysplastic syndrome, therapy related
- AML, not otherwise categorized.

Cytomorphology of AML:

- Round or highly irregular nucleus
- Fine chromatin
- Prominent nucleolus
- Azurophilic granules (sometimes)
- Mature granulocytes (some subtypes)

As with ALL, characteristic features of AML are best seen on Wright–Giemsa-stained preparations (Fig. 10.18). Although azurophilic granules can be present, they are not diagnostic of AML because they are also seen in some cases of ALL. An important finding in many but not all cases of AML is the Auer rod.

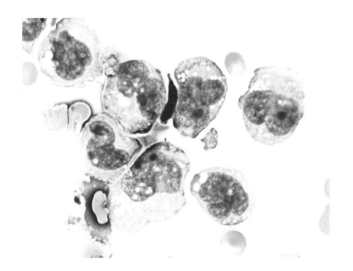

FIG. 10.18. *Acute myeloid leukemia.* In CSF from patients with leukemia, it is usually sufficient simply to identify the presence of blasts; further typing (myeloid vs. lymphoid and their subtypes) is done on peripheral blood and bone marrow biopsy and aspirated material (Wright–Giemsa stain).

This linear structure is a crystallization of azurophilic granules and is pathognomonic of a myeloid disorder. More mature cells such as granulocytes can be present. In evaluating the CSF, it is usually sufficient simply to identify blasts, because definitive diagnosis of ALL or AML and their subtypes depends on the evaluation of the bone marrow aspirate and biopsy.

Chronic Lymphocytic Leukemia

Chronic lymphocytic leukemia (CLL) predominantly affects adults and has a long and protracted clinical course. Despite this, leptomeningeal metastasis is extremely uncommon. The cells of CLL are morphologically indistinguishable from small, mature lymphocytes. It is very important, therefore, to exclude peripheral blood contamination from a traumatic tap: if the sample contains a significant number of red blood cells and the patient is known to have circulating leukemic cells at the time of specimen procurement, the CSF sample is essentially noncontributory. Even if red blood cells are scant or absent, immunophenotyping of the lymphoid cells must be performed to exclude meningitis due to a compromised immune system.

Myeloproliferative Neoplasms

The myeloproliferative neoplasms are clonal hematopoietic stem cell disorders characterized by a bone marrow proliferation of granulocytic, erythroid, or megakaryocytic cells. Clinically heterogeneous, they include chronic myelogenous leukemia, chronic neutrophilic leukemia, chronic eosinophilic leukemia, polycythemia vera, primary myelofibrosis, essential thrombocythemia, mastocytosis, and myeloproliferative neoplasm, unclassifiable. During the chronic phase, the neoplastic cells are minimally invasive, confined to bone marrow, blood, liver, and spleen, and they virtually never involve the CSF. Unfortunately, most patients eventually develop "blast crisis", a transformation to acute leukemia that is almost always fatal, involving the CNS in some patients. As with other leukemias, opportunistic infections are common and must be suspected when a specimen is examined.

Malignant Lymphoma

Leptomeningeal metastasis occurs in 5–10% of patients with non-Hodgkin lymphoma, either at presentation, at a later point during the disease course, or at relapse. Leptomeningeal involvement is more common than parenchymal brain involvement by lymphoma. Some histologic types have a higher incidence of CNS involvement than others. Diffuse large B-cell, lymphoblastic, Burkitt, and Burkitt-like lymphomas have an especially high affinity for the CNS. On the other hand, some lymphomas like Hodgkin lymphoma and small lymphocytic lymphoma are almost never seen in CSF. Patients with leptomeningeal metastasis due to lymphoma have a higher frequency of cranial nerve signs and symptoms.

Cytomorphology of lymphoma in CSF:

- Dispersed cells
- Larger than normal lymphocytes
- Irregular nuclear contours
- Abnormal chromatin
- Prominent nucleolus

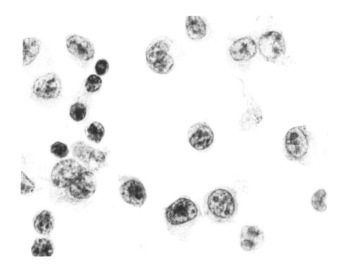

FIG. 10.19. *Diffuse large B-cell lymphoma.* Tumor cells are dispersed as isolated cells with irregular nuclei, coarsely textured chromatin, and scant to abundant cytoplasm. Pyknosis and karyorrhexis are common and can be prominent. A few small benign lymphocytes are present (Papanicolaou stain).

Typically, the CSF shows a monomorphous population of highly atypical cells, with perhaps only a small percentage of normal lymphocytes (Fig. 10.19). In some cases, however, the lymphoma cells are a minority of the total cell population.

The differential diagnosis is a reactive lymphocytosis caused by meningitis. A reactive lymphocytosis is composed of a heterogeneous population of small, mature lymphocytes as well as larger, activated, so-called "atypical" lymphocytes. This distinction is not always straightforward.

Because lymphomas have many different appearances, comparison with a previous biopsy of a lymph node or other site is helpful. In some cases, definitive diagnosis is not possible without lymphoid marker studies. These can be performed on duplicate air-dried cytospins stained with antibodies against a pan B-cell marker (e.g., CD20), a pan T-cell marker (e.g., CD3), and kappa and lambda immunoglobulin light chains (Fig. 10.20a–c). Alternatively, fluid

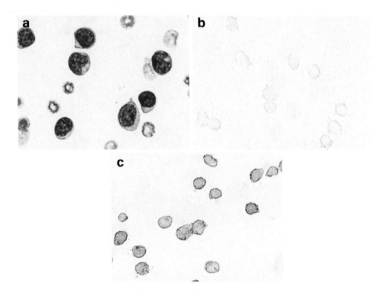

FIG. 10.20. *Follicular lymphoma.* The malignant cells are relatively small and have irregular nuclear contours. The cells show monotypic expression of immunoglobulin light chains. (**a**) Wright–Giemsa stain, (**b**) kappa, and (**c**) lambda.

can be sent fresh for flow cytometric assessment of lymphocyte surface markers. When used selectively, successful results are obtained by flow cytometry in up to 75% of cases. In combination with cytology in the evaluation of atypical lymphoid cells in CSF, flow cytometry improves sensitivity for malignancy. Most reactive and inflammatory fluids are composed primarily of T-cells (Lyme disease is an exception), whereas the great majority of lymphomas that involve the CNS are B-cell neoplasms. Thus, a predominantly B-cell proliferation in CSF is highly suspicious for lymphoma; the diagnosis can be established by demonstrating light chain restriction (predominance of either kappa or lambda expression). The polymerase chain reaction is useful in selected cases and can be performed on archival as well as fresh CSF samples.

Primary CNS Tumors

CSF cytology is an important test for documenting leptomeningeal metastasis of a primary CNS tumor, either at the time of presenta-

TABLE 10.2. Clinical features of primary CNS tumors that spread via CSF pathways.

Tumor	Predominant age	Preferred location(s)
Medulloblastoma	Children	Cerebellum
Glioblastoma	Adults	Cerebral hemispheres
Ependymoma	Children and adolescents	Fourth ventricle (children); spinal cord (adults)
Choroid plexus tumors	Children	Ventricles (most common = fourth)
Pineoblastoma	Children	Pineal gland
Germ cell tumors	Children and adolescents	Pineal, suprasellar regions
Atypical teratoid/ rhabdoid tumor	Infants and children	Cerebellum, brainstem, cerebral hemispheres
Primary CNS lymphoma	Adults	Cerebral hemispheres, cerebellum, brain stem, spinal cord

tion or recurrence. Certain CNS tumors have a greater predilection for involving the leptomeninges than others. These include medulloblastoma, ependymoma, germinoma, pineoblastoma, primitive neuroectodermal tumors (PNETs), atypical teratoid/rhabdoid tumor, choroid plexus tumors, astrocytomas and glioblastomas, and primary CNS lymphomas. The clinical features of some of these are summarized in Table 10.2.

Primary CNS Lymphoma

Primary CNS lymphoma represents between 4% and 15% of all primary CNS tumors. It occurs in both immunocompetent and immunocompromised patients. Epstein–Barr virus is detected in most primary CNS lymphomas in immunocompromised patients and almost never in those arising in immunocompetent individuals. Diffuse large B-cell lymphoma is the most common type; the indolent small cell lymphomas and lymphomas of T-cell phenotype occur much less frequently. In most patients with primary CNS lymphoma, the tumor involves the brain parenchyma, with or without leptomeningeal involvement. But about 8% of cases involve the leptomeninges only ("primary leptomeningeal lymphoma").

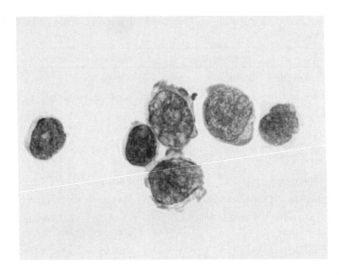

FIG. 10.21. *Primary CNS lymphoma.* Four large, atypical lymphoid cells are present in this field. (Two benign lymphocytes are smaller, with darker nuclei.) In some cases of primary CNS lymphoma, the malignant B-cells are outnumbered by small reactive T-cells, and the findings mimic aseptic meningitis. In this case there was a strong clinical suspicion of malignancy because the patient had cranial nerve findings (diplopia and facial droop). A portion of the sample was sent for flow cytometry, which showed immunoglobulin light chain restriction by the large cells (Wright-Giemsa stain).

CSF cytology is positive in one-third of patients. The diagnosis is difficult because in some cases the large atypical cells are outnumbered by small reactive T-cells, thus mimicking the appearance of an aseptic meningitis (Fig. 10.21). Flow cytometric analysis can be helpful by proving clonality and is highly sensitive: the technique can detect malignant cells that represent as few as 2% of the total cell population. It is not practical to do flow cytometric analysis on all samples that show a lymphocytic pleocytosis, but flow cytometry should be considered in patients with suspicious clinical symptoms. Localized neurologic signs such as cranial nerve palsies are common in patients with primary CNS lymphoma and rare in patients with aseptic meningitis.

Medulloblastoma

Medulloblastoma is a poorly differentiated small cell tumor of uncertain histogenesis that arises in the cerebellum. It is predominantly a disease of children but is sometimes seen in adults. It tends to invade the adjacent fourth ventricle and/or meninges; approximately 25% of patients with medulloblastoma have positive CSF cytology. At autopsy, leptomeningeal involvement is discovered in more than 50% of cases. Morphologically identical tumors in the cerebrum or suprasellar region are called supratentorial primitive neuroectodermal tumors (PNETs).

Cytomorphology of medulloblastoma (Fig. 10.22):

- Small- to medium-sized cells
- Hyperchromatic nucleus
- Scant cytoplasm
- Nucleolus may be prominent
- Nuclear molding

Differential diagnosis of medulloblastoma:

- Poorly preserved lymphocytes
- Germinal matrix
- Small cell carcinoma
- Pineoblastoma
- Neuroblastoma
- Retinoblastoma
- Anaplastic ependymoma

When clusters of small cells are seen in a neonate, especially one born prematurely, they most likely represent cells of germinal matrix origin (see Fig. 10.6). These cells mimic a poorly differentiated small cell malignancy like medulloblastoma. Clinical correlation is very important: the possibility of benign cells of germinal matrix origin should be considered in all neonates with hydrocephalus and in premature infants with intraventricular hemorrhage. In cases associated with hemorrhage, hemosiderin-

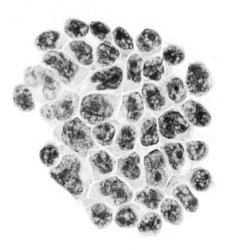

FIG. 10.22. *Medulloblastoma*. The tumor cells are small, with hyperchromatic, irregular nuclei and scant cytoplasm. Nuclear molding is prominent (Papanicolaou stain).

laden macrophages are numerous. Morphologically, medulloblastoma cells are indistinguishable from those of other anaplastic small cell tumors like small cell carcinoma of the lung, but clinical and radiographic findings help in establishing the diagnosis. Anaplastic ependymoma of the fourth ventricle may be clinically and cytologically impossible to distinguish from medulloblastoma however.

Astrocytomas and Glioblastoma

This group of tumors is the most commonly encountered primary CNS malignancy in adults. They arise from astrocytes, the supporting cells of the CNS, and are divided into diffusely infiltrating astrocytomas, pilocytic astrocytoma (WHO grade I), and a few other rare types. Diffusely infiltrating astrocytomas are further subclassified as diffuse astrocytomas (WHO grade II), anaplastic astrocytomas (WHO grade III), and glioblastoma (WHO grade

IV), based on the degree of nuclear pleomorphism, necrosis, and vascular proliferation. These tumors can arise virtually anywhere in the CNS (cerebrum, cerebellum, brain stem, and spinal cord), and all types can spread to the ventricles and subarachnoid space.

Glioblastoma, the highest grade astrocytoma, is the most common of all brain tumors. It comprises 12–15% of all intracranial tumors and more than half of all astrocytic neoplasms. *Pilocytic astrocytoma* is a circumscribed, slowly growing, often cystic tumor that arises in children and young adults. Subarachnoid space involvement is a characteristic feature of pilocytic astrocytomas, and CSF is positive in 11% of patients in whom it is examined, but dissemination along CSF pathways is uncommon. An uncommon type of astrocytic neoplasm, *gliomatosis cerebri*, presents as a diffuse astrocytic proliferation without an obvious tumor mass. It often spreads to involve the subarachnoid space, and CSF examination is useful in establishing a diagnosis.

Cytomorphology of anaplastic astrocytoma and glioblastoma:

- Large pleomorphic cells, or
- Smaller, anaplastic cells with hyperchromatic nuclei

Anaplastic astrocytomas and glioblastomas appear as isolated cells and small clusters. They have hyperchromatic, highly pleomorphic nuclei with coarse chromatin, irregular nuclear outlines, and prominent nucleoli (Fig. 10.23).

Pilocytic astrocytomas appear in CSF as isolated cells or clusters. The isolated cells have long, hairlike cytoplasmic processes, and clustered cells appear epithelioid, often with finely textured chromatin and cobweb-like cytoplasm.

Ependymoma

Ependymomas arise from the lining cells of the ventricles and can occur anywhere in the CNS, but the fourth ventricle and spinal cord are the most common sites. Although more common in children and adolescents, they are also seen in adults. Histologically, ependymomas are considered WHO grade II neoplasms and are comprised of monomorphic cells that form perivascular pseudorosettes and ependymal rosettes, and mitoses are rare. The prognosis is poor because their location makes them inoperable. Of the patients who undergo CSF cytologic examination, 11% have either suspicious or positive cytology. Clinically significant leptomeningeal metastasis is uncommon, however, most likely because of the inability of the seedlings to adhere and proliferate.

The *myxopapillary ependymoma* is a slowly growing, WHO grade I tumor with a favorable prognosis. It accounts for 13% of all ependymomas, has a predilection for young adults, and is virtually always located at the terminal end of the spinal cord. *Anaplastic ependymomas* represent the other end of the spectrum of ependymomas. Considered WHO grade III tumors, anaplastic ependymomas are poorly differentiated, with brisk mitotic activity.

Cytomorphology of ependymomas:

- Isolated cells or small groups
- Round, eccentrically placed nucleus

The appearance of ependymoma cells in CSF depends on the histologic subtype. The cells of the usual type of ependymoma are cuboidal or columnar (Fig. 10.24), with a round or oval, bland nucleus and a moderate amount of cytoplasm. They can be difficult to distinguish from benign ependymal cells. In patients with a tanycytic ependymoma, CSF samples show bipolar cells with long, hairlike glial processes. Anaplastic ependymomas are cytologically indistinguishable from medulloblastomas.

Oligodendroglioma

This tumor of oligodendrocytes is more common in adults but is also seen in children. The great majority occur in the cerebral hemisphere. Spread to the CSF can be either rapid and fatal or chronic and sustained. The tumor is composed of uniform polygonal cells with round nuclei. In tissue sections there is a pronounced perinuclear cytoplasmic clearing that imparts a characteristic "fried egg" appearance to the tumor cells. Positive CSF has been reported, but the cytologic features have not been described in depth.

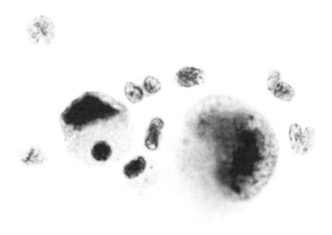

FIG. 10.23. *Glioblastoma.* The tumor cells are highly pleomorphic, with hyperchromatic nuclei and abundant cytoplasm (Papanicolaou stain).

Cytomorphology of oligodendroglioma:

* Uniform round cells
* Distinct cell outlines
* Abundant clear cytoplasm
* Round nucleus
* Fine chromatin
* Prominent nucleolus

Atypical Teratoid/Rhabdoid Tumor

The atypical teratoid/rhabdoid tumor (ATRT) is a newly described CNS tumor of unknown histogenesis that predominantly affects infants and children. One-third of patients have leptomeningeal metastasis at presentation. Histologically and cytologically, the tumor contains rhabdoid cells: medium-sized to large cells with a round, eccentrically placed nucleus and a prominent nucleolus. The cytoplasm is homogeneous and may contain a large, poorly

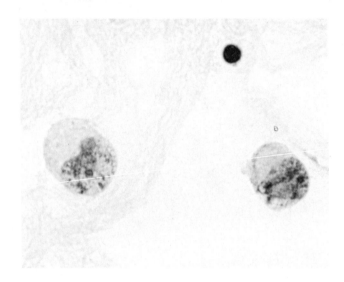

FIG. 10.24. *Ependymoma.* The tumor cells have a round, eccentrically placed nucleus (Papanicolaou stain).

defined, dense, inclusion-like structure that pushes aside the nucleus (Fig. 10.25). Binucleated cells can be seen. Two-thirds of cases have a poorly differentiated small cell component that resembles medulloblastoma cells in CSF. ATRT cells are immunoreactive for epithelial membrane antigen and vimentin, and they may express smooth muscle actin, GFAP, neurofilament protein, and keratin.

Choroid Plexus Tumors

Tumors of the choroid plexus account for 0.5–0.6% of intracranial tumors. Predominantly seen in children, they also occur in adults. The fourth ventricle is the most common location, followed by the lateral ventricles and the third ventricle. The great majority are cytologically benign choroid plexus papillomas. Histologically, the tumors are papillary, composed of a fibrovascular core covered by a single layer of cuboidal or columnar epithelium.

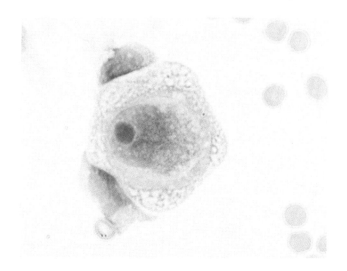

FIG. 10.25. *Atypical teratoid/rhabdoid tumor.* This large rhabdoid cell has a dense cytoplasmic "body" that pushes the nucleus to an eccentric position. Two monocytes and some red blood cells are also present (Wright-Giemsa stain).

Cytomorphology – choroid plexus papilloma:

- Large clusters
- Uniform cuboidal cells
- Round nucleus

The individual cells of a choroid plexus papilloma can be indistinguishable from normal choroid plexus or ependymal cells. When present in abundance and in large clusters, the diagnosis of a papilloma is suggested.

Choroid plexus carcinomas are rare, arising almost exclusively in infants and children. Their existence in adults has been questioned.

Cytomorphology – choroid plexus carcinoma:

- Single cells or clusters
- Pleomorphic nuclei
- Prominent nucleolus
- Indistinguishable from adenocarcinoma

In adults, a metastasis from an occult lung adenocarcinoma must be excluded clinically before the diagnosis can be considered.

Pineal Tumors

The pineal gland is a small, midline structure whose precise function is not known. Pineal tumors are rare, accounting for 0.4–1% of intracranial tumors. More than half of the tumors that arise here are germ cell tumors (discussed below). The rest arise from astrocytes or from specialized neurons called pinealocytes. Tumors of pinealocytic origin affect children more often than adults. They are subclassified as pineocytomas, pineoblastomas, and pineal parenchymal tumors of intermediate differentiation. Pineoblastomas commonly spread to the CSF; in a study of 11 cases, all showed leptomeningeal involvement at autopsy. Pineoblastoma is morphologically indistinguishable from medulloblastoma.

Pineocytomas are typically localized neoplasms that do not metastasize. Although aggressive behavior has been described, some authors question whether these aggressive tumors might have been misclassified.

Germ Cell Tumors

Germ cell neoplasms in the brain arise from primordial germ cells that migrated to the CNS, particularly to the pineal and suprasellar areas. The entire spectrum of testicular and ovarian germ cell tumors can be seen. The most common is the germinoma, histologically identical to the testicular seminoma and the ovarian dysgerminoma and equally radiosensitive. It occurs most commonly in children and young adults, and is more common in males than females. It is likely to infiltrate ventricles and meninges and spread via the CSF. In one study, two of seven patients had positive cytology on CSF examination. Serum and/or CSF elevations of alpha-fetoprotein, beta-HCG, and placental alkaline phosphatase are considered strong presumptive evidence in patients suspected of harboring a CNS germ cell tumor.

Cytomorphology – germinoma:

- Isolated cells
- Large, round nucleus
- Prominent nucleolus
- Moderate amount of cytoplasm

Other types of germ cell tumors, including embryonal carcinoma, endodermal sinus tumor, teratoma, choriocarcinoma, and various combinations of these tumors can also occur, and can be identified in CSF. Choriocarcinomas are highly chemosensitive, and early diagnosis is essential for the prompt institution and success of therapy.

Other Tumors of the CNS

Some of the very common tumors of the CNS rarely spread by CSF pathways and are therefore rarely diagnosed by CSF cytology. Meningiomas constitute 14% of intracranial tumors and almost all are benign. Their spread by means of CSF is extremely uncommon and probably not distinguishable by cytologic methods. Pituitary adenomas represent up to 25% of intracranial tumors. Most are benign, but a small percentage spread to the CSF. In a study of 20 cases, the CSF was positive in both of the patients whose tumors behaved aggressively. Exfoliated cells are arranged in clusters that mimic metastatic adenocarcinoma.

Selected References

Ahmed SV, Jayawarna C, Jude E. Post lumbar puncture headache: diagnosis and management. Postgrad Med J. 2006;82(973):713–6.

Aichner F, Schuler G. Primary leptomeningeal melanoma: diagnosis by ultrastructural cytology of cerebrospinal fluid and cranial computed tomography. Cancer. 1982;50:1751–6.

Balhuizen JC, Bots GT, Schaberg A, et al. Value of cerebrospinal fluid cytology for the diagnosis of malignancies in the central nervous system. J Neurosurg. 1978;48:747–53.

Barshes N, Demopoulos A, Engelhard HH. Anatomy and physiology of the leptomeninges and CSF space. Cancer Treat Res. 2005;125:1–16.

Bigner SH, Johnston WW. The diagnostic challenge of tumors manifested initially by the shedding of cells into cerebrospinal fluid. Acta Cytol. 1984;28:29–36.

Bigner SH, Johnston WW. Cytopathology of the central nervous system. Chicago: American Society of Clinical Pathologists Press; 1994.

Bonnín JM, Garcia JH. Primary malignant non-Hodgkin's lymphoma of the central nervous system. Pathol Annu. 1987;22:353–75.

Boogerd W, Vroom TM. Meningeal involvement as the initial symptom of B cell chronic lymphocytic leukemia. Eur Neurol. 1986;25:461–4.

Boogerd W, Vroom TM, Van Heerde P, et al. CSF cytology versus immunocytochemistry in meningeal carcinomatosis. J Neurol Neurosurg Psychiatry. 1988;51:142–5.

Borowitz MJ, DiGiuseppe JA. Acute lymphoblastic leukemia. In: Knowles DM, editor. Neoplastic hematopathology. Philadelphia: Lippincott Williams & Wilkins; 2001. p. 1643–65.

Borowitz M, Bigner SH, Johnston WW. Diagnostic problems in the cytologic evaluation of cerebrospinal fluid for lymphoma and leukemia. Acta Cytol. 1981;25:665–74.

Breuer AC, Tyler HR, Marzewski DJ, et al. Radicular vessels are the most probable source of needle induced blood in lumbar puncture: significance for the thrombocytopenic cancer patient. Cancer. 1982;49: 2168–72.

Brogi E, Cibas ES. Cytologic detection of Toxoplasma gondii tachyzoites in cerebrospinal fluid. Am J Clin Pathol. 2000;114:951–5.

Browne TJ, Goumnerova LC, De Girolami U, et al. Cytologic features of pilocytic astrocytoma in cerebrospinal fluid specimens. Acta Cytol. 2004;48(1):3–8.

Brunning RD. Acute myeloid leukemia. In: Knowles DM, editor. Neoplastic hematopathology. Philadelphia: Lippincott Williams & Wilkins; 2001. p. 1667–715.

Buchino JJ, Mason KG. Choroid plexus papilloma: report of a case with cytologic differential diagnosis. Acta Cytol. 1992;36:95–7.

Chamberlain MC. Neoplastic meningitis. Semin Neurol. 2004;24(4): 363–74.

Chan TY, Parwani AV, Levi AW, et al. Mollaret's meningitis: cytopathologic analysis of fourteen cases. Diagn Cytopathol. 2003;28(5): 227–31.

Chen KT, Moseley D. Cartilage cells in cerebrospinal fluid. Arch Pathol Lab Med. 1990;114:212.

Chhieng DC, Elgert P, Cohen JM, et al. Cytology of primary central nervous system neoplasms in cerebrospinal fluid specimens. Diagn Cytopathol. 2002;26(4):209–12.

Csako G, Chandra P. Bronchioloalveolar carcinoma presenting with meningeal carcinomatosis: cytologic diagnosis in cerebrospinal fluid. Acta Cytol. 1986;30:653–6.

D'Andrea AD, Packer RJ, Rorke LB, et al. Pineocytomas of childhood: a reappraisal of natural history and response to therapy. Cancer. 1987;59:1353–7.

Davies SF, Gormus BJ, Yarchoan R, et al. Cryptococcal meningitis with false-positive cytology in the CSF: use of T-cell rosetting to exclude meningeal lymphoma. JAMA. 1978;22:2369–70.

De Reuck J, Vanderdonckt P. Choroid plexus and ependymal cells in CSF cytology. Clin Neurol Neurosurg. 1986;88:177–9.

De Reuck J, Vanderdonckt P, de Bleecker J, et al. Mitotic activity in cerebrospinal fluid cells. Clin Neurol Neurosurg. 1988;90:117–9.

DeAngelis LM, Boutros D. Leptomeningeal metastasis. Cancer Invest. 2005;23(2):145–54.

DeGirolami U, Schmidek H. Clinicopathological study of 53 tumors of the pineal region. J Neurosurg. 1973;9:455–62.

Dufour H. Méningite sarcomateuse diffuse avec envahissement de la Moelle et des Racines: cytologie positive et spéciale du liquide céphalorachidien. Rev Neurol. 1904;12:104–6.

Duma RJ, Ferrell HW, Nelson EC, et al. Primary amebic meningoencephalitis. N Engl J Med. 1969;281:1315–23.

Dyken PR. Cerebrospinal fluid cytology: practical clinical usefulness. Neurology. 1975;25:210–7.

Enting RH. Leptomeningeal neoplasia: epidemiology, clinical presentation, CSF analysis and diagnostic imaging. Cancer Treat Res. 2005;125:17–30.

Finn WG, Peterson LC, James C, et al. Enhanced detection of malignant lymphoma in cerebrospinal fluid by multiparameter flow cytometry. Am J Clin Pathol. 1988;110:3416.

Fischer JR, Davey DD, Gulley ML, et al. Blast-like cells in cerebrospinal fluid of neonates: possible germinal matrix origin. Am J Clin Pathol. 1989;91:255–8.

Fishman RA. Cerebrospinal fluid in diseases of the nervous system. 2nd ed. Philadelphia: WB Saunders; 1992.

French CA, Dorfman DM, Shaheen G, et al. Diagnosing lymphoproliferative disorders involving the cerebrospinal fluid: increased sensitivity using flow cytometric analysis. Diagn Cytopathol. 2000;23:369–74.

Gétaz EP, Miller GJ. Spinal cord involvement in chronic lymphocytic leukemia. Cancer. 1979;43:1858–61.

Gindhart TD, Tsukahara YC. Cytologic diagnosis of pineal germinoma in cerebrospinal fluid and sputum. Acta Cytol. 1979;23:341–6.

Glantz MJ, Cole BF, Glantz LK, et al. Cerebrospinal fluid cytology in patients with cancer: minimizing false-negative results. Cancer. 1998;82(4):733–9.

Glass JP, Melamed M, Chernik NL, et al. Malignant cells in cerebrospinal fluid (CSF): the meaning of a positive CSF cytology. Neurology. 1979;29:1369–75.

Gondos B, King EB. Cerebrospinal fluid cytology: diagnostic accuracy and comparison of different techniques. Acta Cytol. 1976;20:542–7.

Granter SR, Doolittle MH, Renshaw AA. Predominance of neutrophils in the cerebrospinal fluid of AIDS patients with cytomegalovirus radiculopathy. Am J Clin Pathol. 1996;105:364–6.

Gupta PK, Gupta PC, Roy S, et al. Herpes simplex encephalitis, cerebrospinal fluid cytology studies: two case reports. Acta Cytol. 1972;16: 563–5.

Hajdu SI, Ashton PR, Carter D, et al. Diagnostic cytology seminar. Acta Cytol. 1982;26:874–6.

Health and Public Policy Committee, American College of Physicians. The diagnostic spinal tap. Ann Intern Med. 1986;104:880–5.

Herrick MK, Rubinstein LJ. The cytological differentiating potential of pineal parenchymal neoplasms (true pinealomas): a clinicopathological study of 28 tumors. Brain. 1979;102:289–320.

Jaffe ES, Harris NL, Stein M, et al., editors. World Health Organization classification of tumours. Pathology and genetics of tumours and haematopoietic and lymphoid tissues. Lyon: IARC Press; 2001.

Jaffey PB, Varma SK, DeMay RM, et al. Blast-like cells in the cerebrospinal fluid of young infants: further characterization of clinical setting, morphology, and origin. Am J Clin Pathol. 1996;105:544–7.

Jereb B, Reid A, Ahuja RK. Patterns of failure in patients with medulloblastoma. Cancer. 1982;50:2941–7.

Kamiya M, Tateyama H, Fujiyoshi Y, et al. Cerebrospinal fluid cytology in immature teratoma of the central nervous system: a case report. Acta Cytol. 1991;35:757–60.

Kaplan JG, DeSouza TG, Farkash A, et al. Leptomeningeal metastases: comparison of clinical features and laboratory data of solid tumors, lymphomas and leukemias. J Neurooncol. 1990;9(3):225–9.

Kim K, Greenblatt SH, Robinson MG. Choroid plexus carcinoma: report of a case with cytopathologic differential diagnosis. Acta Cytol. 1985;29:846–9.

Kjeldsberg CR, Knight JA. Body fluids: laboratory examination of amniotic, cerebrospinal, seminal, serous, and synovial fluids. 3rd ed. Chicago: American Society of Clinical Pathologists Press; 1993.

Kleihues P, Cavenee W, editors. Pathology and genetics of tumours of the nervous system. Lyon: IARC Press; 2000.

Kruskall MS, Carter SR, Ritz LP. Contamination of cerebrospinal fluid by vertebral bone marrow cells during lumbar puncture. N Engl J Med. 1983;308(12):697–700.

Kuberski T. Eosinophils in the cerebrospinal fluid. Ann Intern Med. 1979;91:70–5.

Lachance DH, O'Neill BP, Macdonald DR, et al. Primary leptomeningeal lymphoma: report of 9 cases, diagnosis with immunocytochemical analysis, and review of the literature. Neurology. 1991;41(1):95–100.

Leiman G, Klein C, Berry AV. Cells of nucleus pulposus in cerebrospinal fluid. A case report. Acta Cytol. 1980;24:347–9.

Li CY, Witzig TE, Phyliky RL, et al. Diagnosis of B-cell non-Hodgkin's lymphoma of the central nervous system by immunocytochemical analysis of cerebrospinal fluid lymphocytes. Cancer. 1986;57:737–44.

Liepman MK, Votaw ML. Meningeal leukemia complicating chronic lymphocytic leukemia. Cancer. 1981;47:2482–4.

Ludwin SK, Conley FK. Malignant meningioma metastasizing through the cerebrospinal pathways. J Neurol Neurosurg Psychiatry. 1975;38:136–42.

Mattu R, Sorbara L, Filie AC, et al. Utilization of polymerase chain reaction on archival cytologic material: a comparison with fresh material with special emphasis on cerebrospinal fluids. Mod Pathol. 2004;17(10):1295–301.

Meyer RJ, Ferreira PP, Cuttner J, et al. Central nervous system involvement at presentation in acute granulocytic leukemia: a prospective cytocentrifuge study. Am J Med. 1980;68:691–4.

Miller RR, Lin F, Mallonee MM. Cytologic diagnosis of gliomatosis cerebri. Acta Cytol. 1981;25:37–9.

Morrison C, Shah S, Flinn IW. Leptomeningeal involvement in chronic lymphocytic leukemia. Cancer Pract. 1998;6(4):223–8.

Naylor B. The cytologic diagnosis of cerebrospinal fluid. Acta Cytol. 1964;8:141–9.

NCCLS. Nongynecologic cytologic specimens: collection and cytopreparatory techniques; Approved guideline. NCCLS document GP23-A. Wayne: NCCLS; 1999.

Nolan CP, Abrey LE. Leptomeningeal metastases from leukemias and lymphomas. Cancer Treat Res. 2005;125:53–69.

Nuckols JD, Liu K, Burchette J, et al. Primary central nervous system lymphomas: a 30 year experience at a single institution. Mod Pathol. 1999;12:1167–73.

Ogilvy KM, Jakubowski J. Intracranial dissemination of pituitary adenomas. J Neurol Neurosurg Psychiatry. 1973;36:199–205.

Packer RJ, Siegel KR, Sutton LN, et al. Leptomeningeal dissemination of primary central nervous system tumors of childhood. Ann Neurol. 1985;18:217–21.

Page R, Doshi B, Sharr MM. Primary intracranial choriocarcinoma. J Neurol Neurosurg Psychiatry. 1986;49:93–5.

Prayson RA, Fischler DF. Cerebrospinal fluid: an 11-year experience with 5951 specimens. Arch Pathol Lab Med. 1998;122:47–57.

Price RA, Johnson WW. The central nervous system in childhood leukemia: I. The arachnoid. Cancer. 1973;31:520–33.

Qian X, Cibas ES, Goumnerova L, et al. Cerebrospinal fluid findings in patients with ependymal neoplasms: a bi-institutional retrospective study of 50 cases. Acta Cytol. 2003;47:826–7.

Quincke H. Die Lumbarpunktion des Hydrocephalus. Klin Wochenschr. 1891;28(929–933):965–8.

Ringenberg QS, Francis R, Doll DC. Meningeal carcinomatosis as the presenting manifestation of tumors of unknown origin. Acta Cytol. 1990;34:590–2.

Rogers LR, Duchesneau PM, Nunez C, et al. Comparison of cisternal and lumbar CSF examination in leptomeningeal metastasis. Neurology. 1992;42(6):1239–41.

Rohlfing MB, Barton TK, Bigner SH, et al. Contamination of cerebrospinal fluid specimens with hematogenous blasts in patients with leukemia. Acta Cytol. 1981;25:611–5.

Ross JS, Magro C, Szyfelbein W, et al. Cerebrospinal fluid pleocytosis in aseptic meningitis: cytomorphic and immunocytochemical features. Diagn Cytopathol. 1991;7(5):532–5.

Schmidt P, NeuenJacob E, Blanke M, et al. Primary malignant melanoblastosis of the meninges: clinical, cytologic and neuropathologic findings in a case. Acta Cytol. 1988;32:713–8.

Schwartz JH, Canellos GP, Young RC, et al. Meningeal leukemia in the blastic phase of chronic granulocytic leukemia. Am J Med. 1975;9: 819–28.

Sciarra D, Carter S. Lumbar puncture headache. JAMA. 1952;148:841–2.

Scully RE, Mark EJ, McNeely WF, et al. Case records of the Massachusetts General Hospital. Case 321987. N Engl J Med. 1987;317:366–75.

Shenkier TN. Unusual variants of primary central nervous system lymphoma. Hematol Oncol Clin North Am. 2005;19(4):651–64, vi.

Shibata D, Nichols P, Sherrod A, et al. Detection of occult CNS involvement of follicular small cleaved lymphoma by the polymerase chain reaction. Mod Pathol. 1990;3:71–5.

Stefanko SZ, Talerman A, Mackay WM, et al. Infundibular germinoma. Acta Neurochir. 1979;50:71–8.

Szyfelbein WM, Ross JS. Lyme disease meningopolyneuritis simulating malignant lymphoma. Mod Pathol. 1988;1:464–8.

Takeuchi J, Handa H, Nagata I. Suprasellar germinoma. J Neurosurg. 1978;49:41–8.

Tedder DG, Ashley R, Tyler KL, et al. Herpes simplex virus infection as a cause of benign recurrent lymphocytic meningitis. Ann Intern Med. 1994;121:334–8.

Torzewski M, Lackner K, Bohl J, et al. Integrated cytology of cerebrospinal fluid. New York: Springer; 2008.

Trojanowski JQ, Atkinson B, Lee VM. An immunocytochemical study of normal and abnormal human cerebrospinal fluid with monoclonal antibodies to glial fibrillary acidic protein. Acta Cytol. 1986;30:235–9.

Vardiman JW, Harris NL, Brunning RD. The World Health Organization (WHO) classification of the myeloid neoplasms. Blood. 2002;100(7):2292–302.

Walts AE. Cerebrospinal fluid cytology: selected issues. Diagn Cytopathol. 1992;8:394–408.

Wasserstrom WR, Glass JP, Posner JB. Diagnosis and treatment of leptomeningeal metastases from solid tumors: experience with 90 patients. Cancer. 1982;49:759–72.

Watson CW, Hajdu SI. Cytology of primary neoplasms of the central nervous system. Acta Cytol. 1977;21:40–7.

Wechsler LR, Gross RA, Miller DC. Meningeal gliomatosis with "negative" CSF cytology: the value of GFAP staining. Neurology. 1984;34:1611–5.

Weller PF, Liu LX. Eosinophilic meningitis. Semin Neurol. 1993;13:161–8.

Wertlake PT, Markovits BA, Stellar S. Cytologic evaluation of cerebrospinal fluid with clinical and histologic correlation. Acta Cytol. 1972;6:229–39.

Wynter W. Four cases of tubercular meningitis in which paracentesis of the theca vertebralis was performed for the relief of fluid pressure. Lancet. 1891;1:981–2.

Yamamoto LJ, Tedder DG, Ashley R, et al. Herpes simplex virus type I DNA in cerebrospinal fluid of a patient with Mollaret's meningitis. N Engl J Med. 1991;325:1082–5.

Zeman D, Adam P, Kalistova H, et al. Cerebrospinal fluid cytologic findings in multiple sclerosis. A comparison between patient subgroups. Acta Cytol. 2001;45:51–9.

Index

S.Z. Ali and E.S. Cibas, *Serous Cavity Fluid and Cerebrospinal
Fluid Cytopathology*, Essentials in Cytopathology 10,
DOI 10.1007/ 978-1-4614-1776-7,
© Springer Science+Business Media, LLC 2012